NATURAL DANDRUFF TREATMENTS

Natural Non-Chemical Treatments for Dandruff Psoriasis and Seborrheic Dermatitis~ Dealing with the "Root" of the Problem~ Do You Really Want to Know?"

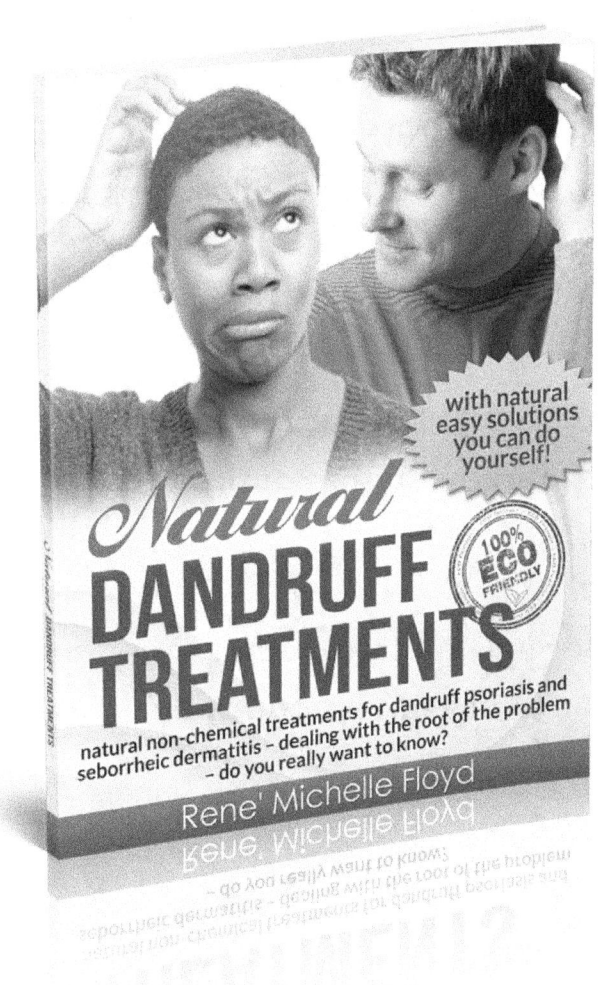

René Michelle Floyd

**Disclaimer: While this information is based on my years of experience and personal knowledge, it is not guaranteed to work on every individual case the same. I, René Michelle Floyd and my company, Beautiful Hair Products (formerly known as Naturally Yours Boutique, Inc.) has provided this book solely for your general information and is in no way intended as your personal medical advice, and should not be depended upon as a substitute for any consultations with your qualified health care practitioner.

Some of the links on the ***resources page (back pages of book)*** are from companies that I'm associated with as an affiliate. If you purchase from them, I will get a small commission. This will not affect you in anyway. You will not be charged at all. I thank you in advance for your support.

Many Thanks

First of all, I'd like to thank my Heavenly Father for blessing me with the power and strength to write this book. It is my intention and purpose to share with others what has worked for me. In doing so, I know this act alone can help someone and save them from hair loss, heart ache and pain.

I am very thankful for my husband Richard, for his patience and belief in me that I would complete this book and finally be satisfied.

To my mom Barbara, I give thanks for lovingly making herself available to me in taking care of our young son while I worked on this, and many other projects.

To ALL of my children, I give thanks. I've spent a lot of time away from you working, working and working. I look forward to making up for some of the lost time.

To all of my clients, friends and family that have shared their thoughts, opinions and answers to surveys, thank you for your input and feedback. It's what has helped me write this book.

My prayer is that someone's life will be enhanced as a result of this work.

Thank you in advance for reading it...now go and *apply* what you read.

Peace.

René Michelle Floyd ~ author

Table of Contents

About René Michelle Floyd

Since the inception of my company, <u>Beautiful Hair Products</u> (formerly

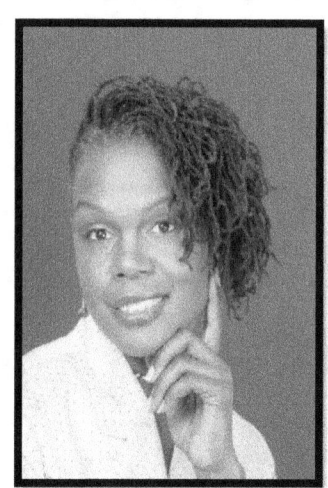

known as Naturally Yours Boutique) in year 2000, my passion has been to focus on the health, care and beauty of naturally kinky coily hair—free of any chemicals which alter its natural texture.

As a little girl, I spent hours combing, brushing and braiding my dolls hair. Once my little sister, Chelsea got old enough, I found myself braiding and styling her hair as well.

Known for my love of *natural solutions* through herbal recipes and remedies, I recommend only the best quality products and solutions available for dry hair and dry scalp.

As an avid researcher, I'm always seeking more knowledge so that I can be more of a resource to my clients, customers and others. I know and understand that the beauty of one's hair is a reflection of their overall health. I am passionate about holistic health. Good health is directly linked to *good hair*.

When we accept and embrace our own natural hair texture and begin patiently nurturing and giving our hair the attention it needs to thrive and grow, we are much happier, confident and fulfilled. There's so much freedom and liberation in accepting the hair that God gave us. No matter how much we try to cover up our own natural hair by wearing wigs, weaves, extension- braids, press-n-curl, bleaching and coloring or perm, our own natural hair and texture will come bursting out, because, it's who we are!"

My Vision

One night I had a vision and a revelation; *LOCs is my style of choice*; it agreed with my hair type, so I started Loc'n my hair. I found that people around me had to adjust to *MY* new hairstyle. It was okay, because I felt this was *my style*.

I wore traditional LOCs (dreadlocks) for 5 years before I cut them out to start over with *Sisterlocks*tm a hairstyle that captured my heart the moment I saw them! I thought, *how beautiful and versatile*.

I had been braid'n, loc'n and twist'n natural hair for many, many years at that point, and had worn natural hair styles most of my life. When I saw Sisterlocks™ I had to have them. These days, my style of choice is *Sisterlocks* tm a natural hair management system originating from Dr. Joann Cornwell. Sisterlocks™ is perfect for individuals with tightly textured hair to take advantage of a wide range of today's hairstyles without having to alter their natural hair texture.

Needless to say, I am very satisfied. I was a Certified Sisterlocks tm Consultant in sunny Southern California for almost 17 years (I am now retired). It was the best profession I could have chosen.

Naturally Yours Boutique Opens Its Doors

NYB (Naturally Yours Boutique) opened its doors to serve the natural hair community in the Inland Empire in Southern California. The need was to have a Professional Natural Hair Care studio to care for and render services for the natural hair needs of that community without having to commute to the big city of Los Angeles just to get their hair done, especially after commuting to work every day of the week.

Creating NYB at the time really was a win-win situation because I was at a cross-road in my life and needed to design a lifestyle for me and my family that would allow me to work and earn a living while being present.

I created my company – Beautiful Hair Products (formerly known as Naturally Yours Boutique, Inc.) on a hope and a dream and have been able to achieve a lot of what I've set out to accomplish. Now my business is expanding and growing and life is good!

I have a lot of gratitude for my God, my journey, my family and my wonderful clients and customers around the world!

The Passion, Mission, Vision and Purpose of René and Beautiful Hair Products

Beautiful Hair Product's Mission is to provide educational information, recommended books, hair techniques, tutorials and natural hair products that promote healthy scalp and beautiful hair.

My Purpose is to provide the world with Natural Hair Care products that encourages ethnic women and men to appreciate and embrace their naturally curly coily beautifully textured hair.

My Vision is to create an atmosphere where people with curlier textured hair will be inspired to change their attitude about accepting and owning their own natural beauty—from head to toe.

My Goal is to help raise the consciousness and self-esteem of our clients and customers around the world and to give them an experience where they will gain confidence and self-empowerment about their natural beauty...from the inside out.

"I have high aspirations for my business and I don't want Beautiful Hair Products to be just another hair business. I want to create a culture where anyone who walks through our doors or visits our website, will experience something they can't find anywhere else." ~ *René Michelle Floyd, Founder*

Why I Wrote Natural Dandruff Treatments

Many times, I was asked if I knew what to do about dry scalp and dandruff. I used to say, "not really," and give the same answers as everybody else; "use this product or that product; this shampoo or that shampoo."

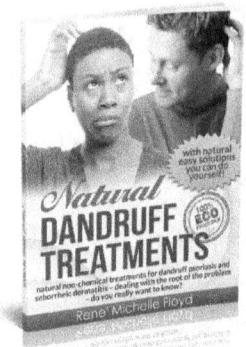

It wasn't until I really started listening with my heart that I decided to do my due diligence and go deeper into my knowledge base. I went on a quest to give accurate and useful (natural) information that would genuinely answer their questions and help bring relief to an aggravating and sometimes challenging medical problem.

I'm very convinced that you don't have to settle for what the norm is and use chemical based products that sometimes perpetuate the dandruff problem in the first place. There are *other alternative products* that are natural and effective and simple. It's been said that *less is more*.

Join me in learning more about the health of the scalp so we all can achieve the beautiful head of hair we deserve. Choose one of the recipe solutions from this book and use it *BEFORE* you use a chemical based product. It is my hope that you find the help and the answers you've been looking for.

Peace,

Rene'

Introduction

As anyone who has ever suffered from dandruff will tell you, it can be a big problem that non-sufferers often don't really understand. And what is not understood by the majority is that while the condition is not necessarily dangerous in health terms, it is definitely harmful to the sufferer in many *other* ways.

Thus, it is understandable that most dandruff sufferers will do whatever they can to get rid of their problem, and in most cases, this is likely to mean turning to commercially produced anti-dandruff products to deal with their problem.

There are plenty of such products on the market today and many of them can be bought across the counter from a standard drug store or pharmacy. Many of the commercial anti-dandruff products are *chemical based*, and as with all products that rely on chemicals for their results, they often have negative and sometimes dangerous side-effects. With this fact in mind, we will be mindful as we explore *other alternative methods.*

DANDRUFF!!!

Doesn't it make sense to consider natural solutions *first* if you suffer from dandruff *before* you use the others? Fortunately, there are quite a number of natural answers to the dandruff question: ***What is dandruff and what causes it?***

The primary purpose of this book is to introduce you to many of the *natural treatments* for dandruff and to share the information provided as you seek for a solution that will work for your situation.

Also included is *new* information about the Malassezia yeast; which of the Malassezia species is connected to dandruff?

I have also included brief descriptions on what (scalp) Psoriasis is; what Seborrheic eczema (Seborrheic dermatitis), Ringworm, Lice and Scabies are as well.

There is also a briefing on *Enema Health* and how keeping the colon clear and flushed out is directly connected to the healing of most ailments and issues in regards to the health of the skin and scalp. Also included, is a section called, **How to give yourself an enema**; this will be your guide in finding healing for your colon.

However, before we get into those topics, we will first examine (1) exactly what dandruff is (2) why people suffer from the problem, and finally (3) natural solutions that will minimize and possibly end skin and scalp problems...forever!

But, before we start anything, let's look at~

FACT: Beautiful hair starts with a healthy scalp

I think many of us miss that realization. In particular when people of color decide to *go natural*- most of us are so excited, but soon become disappointed because we discover that our hair is *hard* and *unmanageable.*

Instead of focusing on the health of our scalp, we focus on what hair products we can buy that will make our hair soft and beautiful.

It is understood culturally that, people of color love to buy and try hair care products...the thought is, if we try this product or that product – this shampoo/conditioner, or that gel, *it* will give us the *look* we want.

What we fail to do when it comes to the products we choose, is to read the labels and understand that there are certain ingredients that are chemical based and does more harm than good to the health of the hair, and especially the health of the scalp.

The key to a healthy scalp is leaving the pores of the skin as clog free as possible. We make the mistake of clogging our scalp with too much gel, waxes and conditioners, laden with petroleum and other clog producing substances.

What those of us who have decided to *go natural* must understand, is that going natural also means going natural in terms of the hair care products we use and the diet and lifestyle we choose. Now, let's take a look at **The 10 Steps to Healthy Scalp & Hair** in detail:

The 10 Steps to Healthy Scalp & Hair...what is your scalp saying?

1. Review your current hair products
2. Remove Malassezia yeast from your scalp
3. Expose your head to sunlight as often as possible
4. Avoid eating spicy foods (too often)
5. Avoid consuming alcohol caffeine and tobacco(as much as possible)
6. Re-evaluate your diet and eating habits
7. Increase your milk and calcium intake
8. Commit to a daily vitamin and mineral regimen
9. Reduce and eliminate stress and anxiety
10. Give yourself daily scalp massages

#1   Review your current hair products

If the products you choose has a lot of alcohol and sulfates and ammonia's which is mostly made up of harsh detergents designed to act as a sudsing agent and to remove dirt and pollution from the hair. A lot of the *popular* anti-dandruff hair products on the market today, are reeking with chemicals that actually break down the protein bonds that provide human hair with its natural texture.

A few chemicals to especially look out for are:

- selenium sulfide
- pyrithione zinc
- Ketoconazole

In extreme cases some of these chemicals can accelerate natural hair loss.

In the chapter-**Commercial Anti-Dandruff Shampoos--Analyzed**, it goes into more detail about this.

#2   Reduce and remove Malassezia yeast

Malassezia (formerly known as Pityrosporum) is a genus of related fungi, classified as yeasts, naturally found on the skin surfaces of many animals including humans. It can cause hypopigmentation.

Hypopigmentation is the loss of skin color. It is caused by melanocyte or melanin depletion, or a decrease in the amino acid tyrosine, which is used by melanocytes to make melanin. Hypopigmentation on the trunk and other locations of the human body becomes an opportunistic for infection.

In the chapter, **what causes dandruff?** goes into more detail on this subject.

#3   Expose your head to sunlight as often as possible

Avoid wearing head gear (caps, hats, scarves, wigs etc.) as much as possible...these items create an environment in which Malassezia yeast thrives in.

#4   Avoid eating spicy foods as much as possible

Eating spicy foods causes sweating in many people and aggravates the problem more.

#5   Avoid consuming alcohol caffeine and tobacco

Substances with alcohol, caffeine and tobacco are toxic in nature and further aggravate the scalp... alcohol and cigarettes worsen psoriasis symptoms, but a number of researchers believe that they may actually cause psoriasis in some patients.

Additionally, alcohol in particular can have very serious side effects when mixed with some psoriasis medications. Alcohol and tobacco may render some medications ineffective. Cigarette smoking increased incidences of psoriasis, as well as decreased rates of recovery from psoriasis in smokers.

#6   Re-evaluate your diet and eating habits

A diet filled with too much sugar, starch and fat can exacerbate your dandruff problem. Your diet is a definite connection to the health of your scalp.

You need to eat more foods rich in minerals and B vitamins. Fruits and vegetables are ideal especially green leafy veggies.
You really are what you eat.

#7   Increase your milk and calcium intake

If you drink milk, whole milk is better because it has your fat soluble vitamins such as vitamin A, K, D and E which are all contained in the milk fat.

Many people have a vitamin D deficiency which is the connection to the inflammatory condition directly related to dandruff.

** There is a section in this book called: **Soymilk: what are the benefits?** The information is very enlightening...Soymilk is a very good source of protein and is rich in minerals, such as magnesium and has more calcium than cow's milk.

#8   Commit to a vitamin and mineral regimen

It goes without saying that our bodies are complex and fearfully and wonderfully made. Our *modern day* microwave type diets have done great harm in its chemical make-up than I'm comfortable with. We must replace the minerals that we lose from partaking in such a poor diet.

Sometimes I get tired of taking my vitamins and minerals and when I don't take them, I feel absolutely lousy. Biotin is wonderful for the scalp and hair. Vitamins and minerals stimulate healthy hair growth and stimulate the scalp. Many vitamins help to fight the yeast on your head which causes scalp issues in the first place.

#9   Reduce and eliminate stress and anxiety

Of course this reality can change your entire lifestyle. By reducing and eliminating stress and anxiety, you will experience a higher quality of life with more vigor and energy and a healthier happier scalp and thriving hair growth.

Slowing down and taking deep breathes can have a wonderful effect on the level of stress you experience. Getting more rest and sleep plays a large part in your amount of new hair growth and scalp health. Your stress and anxiety levels will greatly reduce.

Taking relaxing baths accompanied by some delicious smelling aromatherapy oils will really make a difference.

The preceding suggestions will make the difference in the health of your scalp.

Natural Dandruff Treatments goes into detail about what type of herbs and oils to use for de-stressing and massaging.

#10 Massage your scalp daily

Head massages are great for stimulating blood flow which encourages hair growth.

Choose a recipe solution from this book and use it *BEFORE* you use chemical based commercial products.

If you have tried everything you can think of but are suffering, **keep reading** and choose a recipe solution from this book, *Natural Dandruff Treatments*. Follow the simple recipe and mix the ingredients together and use it at least a couple of months ***BEFORE*** using chemical based products. Patience is a virtue. Give it some time to work for you.

Now, let's examine **what dandruff is**…

PART 1

WHAT IS DANDRUFF?

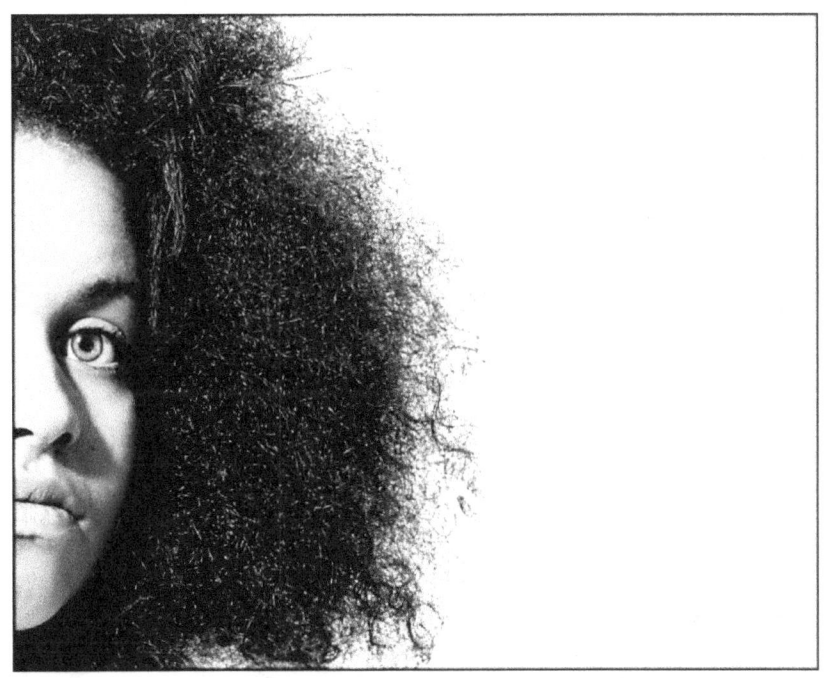

What is Dandruff?

Dandruff is the shedding of dead skin cells from the scalp in either oily

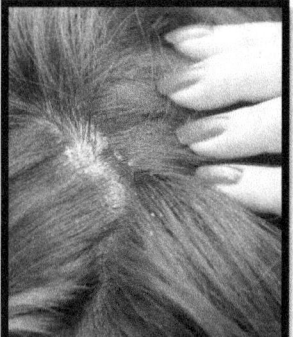

clumps or as dry flakes.

Dandruff is a condition that can be suffered in varying degrees, ranging from extremely mild to severe. Dandruff is a problem that is familiar to many millions of people all over the world.

Procter & Gamble, best known for their commercially produced anti-dandruff shampoos, suggests that perhaps 60% of US citizens will suffer from dandruff at one time or another in their lifetime.

Again, the basic symptom of dandruff is the shedding of dead skin cells from the scalp, which is in fact a process that takes place all of the time for every person. However, the difference between the shedding of dead skin cells for a non-dandruff sufferer and for someone who has the condition is a question of degree.

Shedding - What's Normal and What's Not

In the normal course of events for someone who does not suffer dandruff, the life cycle of average skin cells is somewhere around 28 days. During this period of time, the skin cells are formed within the body before being gradually pushed to the outermost epidermal layer of

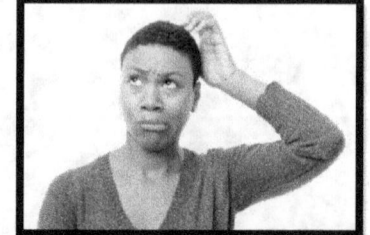

the skin. Once the cells reach the very outer layer of the skin, in contact with the air, they quickly die and are shed by the body.

However, because these dead cells are infinitesimally small, and invisible to the naked eye, and because the number of cells being shed is 'normal', the process is unnoticeable.

On the other hand, in the case of someone who suffers dandruff, the situation is significantly different. In this case, the individual concerned is producing far too many skin cells, with the whole cell production process taking place in something between two and seven days (instead of the normal 28 days). The result is that these cells are shed in oily clumps or as flakes, hence the evidence --dandruff.

Is Dandruff Curable?

In effect, someone who suffers from dandruff is simply showing the visible signs of an exaggerated physiological process, with their body

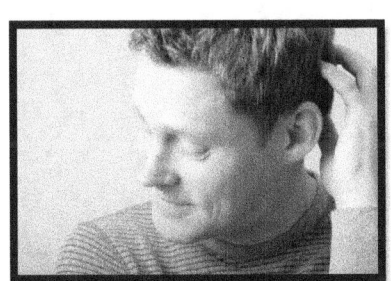

working too quickly to process the job that for a non-dandruff sufferer is something that will not even get noticed.

The shedding of oily clumps or dry flakes of the skin is often accompanied by redness and irritation. So, not only does dandruff look unpleasant to other people, it can also be an unpleasant problem for the sufferer too.

Contrary to popular theory, dandruff does not necessarily imply that your head or your hair is dirty, **nor is the condition contagious**.

It has been said that as a physiological process, dandruff can never be completely cured, only treated-quite to the contrary.

There has been testimony after testimony of people, upon changing their anti-dandruff products and their lifestyle and diet, that they have found the *cure* to their lifelong problem.

Any claims that dandruff cannot be cured is something to be viewed with a good deal of skepticism and doubt.

Once again, dandruff is a condition that can be suffered in varying degrees, ranging from extremely mild to severe.

**In most cases, there is no need to consult the medical profession to deal with a dandruff problem unless it is extreme and serious, or because it is related to some other condition which does necessitate medical attention.

Flaky Scalp – Is Dandruff the Only Cause?

Most people have met someone who suffers from dandruff if they do

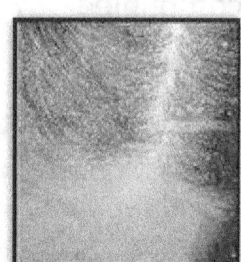

not suffer from the condition themselves. At some time or another, we have all encountered someone with the tell-tale signs of white flakes in their hair and on their shoulders, so most of us are familiar with what dandruff looks like.

However, the white clumps or dry flakes on the shoulders of someone wearing dark clothing do not necessarily indicate a person who suffers from dandruff, because there are other conditions that can cause the skin on the scalp to flake in a similar way.

Some of these conditions might require medical attention or special treatment, so you cannot automatically assume that flaky skin landing on your shoulders immediately tells you that you have dandruff (although dandruff would be by far the most common cause of flaky skin).

Learning to recognize these *other conditions* is valuable, as it should enable you to differentiate between dandruff and something else that might be (or may become) a more serious case and possibly worthy of special medical attention, if necessary.

What is Seborrheic Dermatitis and Eczema -are they related to dandruff?

Seborrheic dermatitis (sometimes called 'Seborrheic eczema') is a form of skin inflammation of unknown cause. The signs and symptoms of Seborrheic eczema/dermatitis include yellowish, oily, scaly patches of

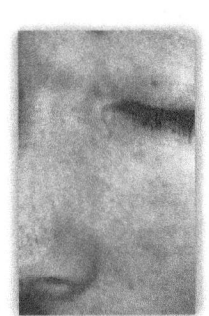

skin that can affect not only the scalp but also other areas of the body including the face, ears and trunk. This is a condition that causes flaking, itchy red skin and is most commonly found in areas of the body where there is the largest number of sebaceous glands.

As these glands are found in hair follicles, it follows

that any part of the body where there is hair present is a place where you might suffer from Seborrheic dermatitis. Often the scaly patches are called 'dandruff' in adults and 'cradle cap' in infants.

Typically, eczema causes skin to become itchy, red and dry—even cracked and leathery.

Eczema is a skin condition caused by inflammation. Atopic dermatitis is the most common of the many types of eczema. While the word **dermatitis means inflammation of the skin**. *Atopic* refers to an allergic tendency, which is often inherited.

Fortunately, while the condition might be visually unpleasant and often causes irritating itching, it is nevertheless harmless. While it is also a condition that can be persistent, it is one that is easily dealt with using either natural means in the majority of cases, or medication if absolutely necessary in the most severe cases.

The good news is the condition is **not contagious** and can't be spread from person to person.

Since the dis-ease makes the skin dry and itchy, lotions and creams are recommended to keep the skin moist and supple. These products are usually applied when the skin is damp, usually after bathing to help the skin retain moisture. Cold (not hot) compresses may also be used to relieve the itching.

One last word of encouragement - usually, **there is *no hair loss*** associated with these conditions.

What is Psoriasis - Can I get it on my Scalp?

In the case of people who suffer from psoriasis, one area of the body that is often affected is the scalp. As the most common form of

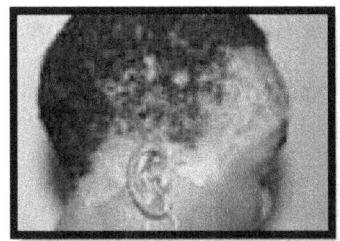

psoriasis (psoriasis vulgaris) is characterized by angry red lesions on the skin with a silvery, flaky upper skin layer, scalp psoriasis will usually cause dead skin flakes to land on your clothes in exactly the same way as dandruff would.

Psoriasis is a medical condition that can vary in degree and severity, with the most severe cases sometimes requiring medical intervention.

And while there are different types of psoriasis, (psoriasis vulgaris, inverse psoriasis, erythro dermic, pustular, guttate, plaque, and psoriatic arthritis) it is a fact that 80% of people who suffer from the condition have psoriasis vulgaris, which would be evident in most sufferers by the angry red lesions or plaques that can appear almost anywhere on the body.

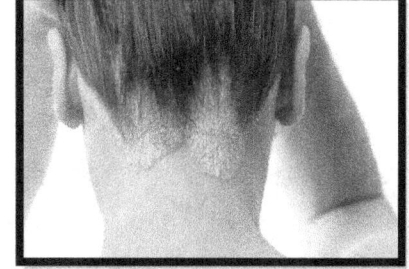

However, the most common place to encounter psoriasis lesions is on the elbows and knees, so if you have skin flakes dropping down from your head as well as red lesions, it is likely that your scalp problem is associated with psoriasis rather than with dandruff.

Scalp psoriasis is a common skin disorder that produces raised, reddish, and often scaly patches. It can appear as one or multiple patches on the scalp, affecting the entire scalp and spreading beyond the scalp to the forehead and to the back of the neck or behind the ears.

Like other types of psoriasis, its exact cause is unknown, however, it is believed to result from an abnormality of the immune system, which causes skin cells to grow too fast and build up as patches or plaque.

Most commonly, however, is people that have scalp psoriasis also have psoriasis on other parts of their body.

Scalp psoriasis can be mild and almost unnoticeable. But it can also be severe and long lasting, causing thick, crusted lesions that affect appearance and self-esteem in some individuals.

Intense itching can interfere with sleep and everyday life. Frequent scratching can lead to skin infections and *potential hair loss.*

Scalp psoriasis is not contagious. It cannot spread from one person to the other. **However, in the most severe cases, seeking medical attention is advisable.

Now, let's take a brief look at 3 different dis-eases:

1. **Ringworm**
2. **Scabies** and
3. **Lice** to see if these three are connected or related at all to dandruff.

Ringworm – Can it Affect My Scalp?

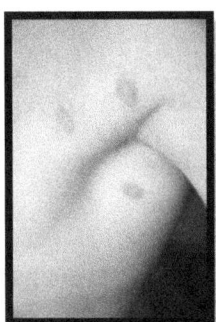 Despite the name, (Tinea capitis) ringworm has nothing to do with worms. It is a fungal infection that leaves ring-shaped, scaly red rashes and patches of *hair loss* on the scalp.

Ringworm is most common in children between the ages of 3 and 7, but can affect adults too. Every person has millions of fungus cells on every part of their body, but for the majority, these fungi cause no problem whatsoever. However, if the skin is damaged in some way, the fungus on the surface can gain access to the body, in which case it is possible that it might cause a fungal infection.

This can happen on any part of the body, including the scalp, so it is entirely possible that from time to time you might suffer a fungal infection that causes the skin cells around the infected area to die in greater numbers than usual. When this happens, you would encounter dandruff-like symptoms as the dead skin cells are shed.

Whether you need to seek medical attention in these circumstances would depend upon the severity of the fungal infection from which you are suffering. However, in the case of fungal infection, it should be evident that something is not quite right because it is most likely to be accompanied by a degree of pain, which is very rare with dandruff.

Ringworm is contagious and can spread from person to person through close contact usually by sharing hats, clothing, scarves, towels and combs and brushes with someone who is infected already. In rare cases, it's possible to catch ringworm from a dog or cat.

Anti-fungal medications taken orally can clear up a ringworm infection, but it may take up to six weeks to four months to do so.

Using an anti-fungal shampoo may help reduce the risk of spreading the infection to family members and classmates. It's important for those individuals who have ringworm to avoid sharing personal items so that they don't pass the infection on to others.

What Are Scabies – is it Related To Dandruff?

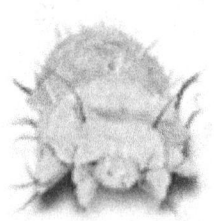 Scabies is an itchy, **highly contagious** skin disease by an infestation of the itch mite – *Sarcoptes scabiel*. The mites are small eight-legged parasite (in contrast to insects, which have six legs). They are tiny, just 1/3 millimeter long, and burrow into the skin to produce intense itching, which tends to be worse at night.

The mites that infest humans are female and are 0.3 mm – 0.4mm long; the males are about half this size. Scabies mites can be seen with a magnifying glass or microscope. The scabies mites crawl but are unable to fly or jump and they move very slowly. They are immobile at temperatures below 20 C, although they may survive for prolonged periods at these temperatures.

Scabies usually is spread by close, intimate contact such as sleeping in the same bed with someone or touching someone who has scabies. After burrowing under the skin, a female mite lays 10 to 25 eggs before she dies. The eggs hatch into larvae 2 to 3 days later. These larvae move to the skin's surface and become adults within about 14 to 17 days. This cycle continues until the mites are killed.

Scabies and dandruff is not really associated because the mites usually burrows where it is rough or wrinkled on your skin, such as elbows, knuckles and knees.

What Are Head Lice?

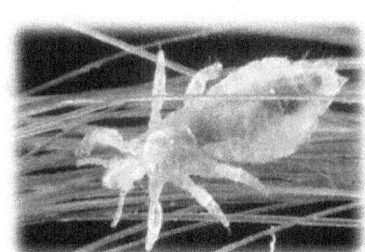

The head louse is a tiny, wingless parasitic insect that lives among human hairs and feeds on extremely small amounts of blood drawn from the scalp. Although they may sound gross, lice (the plural of louse) are a very common problem, especially for kids' ages 3 years to 12 years (girls more often than boys).

Lice aren't dangerous and they don't spread disease, but are **highly contagious** and can just be downright annoying! Their bites may cause a child's scalp to become itchy and inflamed, and persistent scratching may lead to skin irritation and even infection. (kidshealth.org)

Lice and Nits – Not a Pleasant Pet

Although it is perhaps not that easy to believe in this day and age, there are still millions of people (mainly children) all over the world who suffer from head lice. For example, it is believed that anywhere from 6 to 12 million people are treated for head lice in 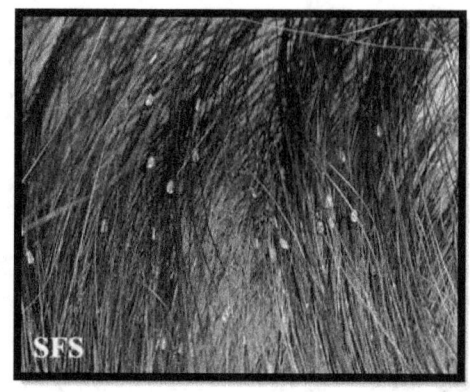 the USA alone every year, while high levels of louse infestation have been reported in countries as diverse as the UK, Australia, Israel, Denmark and Sweden.

And in the case of louse infestation, it is possible that the excoriation (or shedding) of skin cells caused by the lice as they go about their business might cause a condition that appears to be similar to dandruff.

Obviously, having lice is not particularly pleasant, nor is it necessarily healthy as they will bite the host skin four or five times a day to feed and inject saliva into the skin when they do so.

There is a myth that says, people with kinky hair cannot get lice. This is a false myth. *ALL people*, with any texture of hair can get an infestation of lice.

Although head lice are not believed to be carriers of any disease, they are certainly something that you want to get rid of as soon as possible, so if there is any reason to suspect an infestation, you should seek attention as soon as possible.

What Kills Lice?

First off, what kill lice are a few things, including:

- Heat
- Olive oil
- Mayonnaise
- Butter

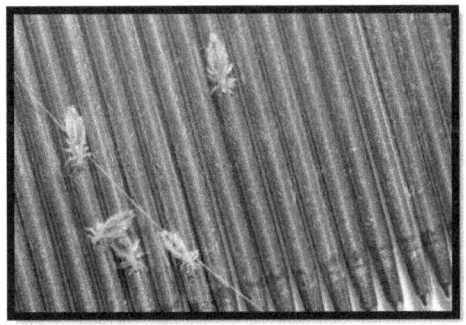

- Vaseline
- Coconut oil
- Garlic
- Tea tree oil

Head lice do not hop, jump or fly. They migrate through direct contact with a person that is currently infested with lice and their belongings.

Pets do not transmit head lice, and poor personal hygiene does not cause an infestation. In fact, head lice prefer clean, healthy heads.

Head lice do not live in, nor spontaneously generate from, the dirt, trees or the air. They live on the human head!

Lice hate dry heat. You can put clothes, hats, towels etc. in a hot dryer for twenty minutes which should kill lice and their eggs.

Lice breathe through holes in their sides. When you cover these holes with olive oil, the lice will die. However, it takes a while for them to die, because head lice can shut down their systems for hours. That's why you need to know exactly how and when to use a smothering program. Olive oil, mayonnaise, butter and Vaseline are smothering agents.

However, unlike olive oil, these substances are difficult to get out of the hair, particularly in the case of Vaseline. Children are often repelled by the smell of butter and mayonnaise and both these substances can turn rancid, and cause problems if children suck on their hair.

Mineral oil (including baby oil) is **not** recommended because it can be harmful to mucous membranes.

Olive Oil is the best smothering agent. It has been lab-tested and found to be effective in killing head lice. Olive oil has few, if any, allergic properties and is relatively inexpensive. The least expensive grade - pumace or restaurant grade - is best. And olive oil can be purchased with food stamps.

Smothering head lice is a safe and effective treatment option, but it can be somewhat complicated. To smother successfully, you have to be persistent and know when and how to apply the smothering agent.

Every successful lice removal program must include manual nit picking. Even if you treat with chemicals and/or olive oil you must also incorporate manual nit picking into your treatment program because nothing has proved successful in killing nits.

Lice lay their eggs close to the scalp. It used to be thought that eggs farther than ½ inch from the scalp were not viable. However, new research indicates that this is not true, especially during warm weather. Therefore, removing all the nits is the only sure way to get an infestation under control. Getting rid of head lice requires perseverance.

For those with kinky dense hair, careful shampooing and cleansing of the scalp and hair is required to kill and clear all nits and lice out the curly hair. For kinky or loc'd hair, dolce your hair with a smothering agent and comb and pick out the nits thoroughly, shampooing several times. If this doesn't work, depending on the severity of the infestation, unfortunately, the curly hair may need to be cut off just to get rid of all the dead critters lodged in the hair.

How to Kill Lice and Nits

- **Comb them out.** Obtain a delousing comb and a bottle of your favorite conditioner. Take a hot shower combing the conditioner through your hair and rinsing the comb and the tips of your hair throughout to wash any lice down the drain.

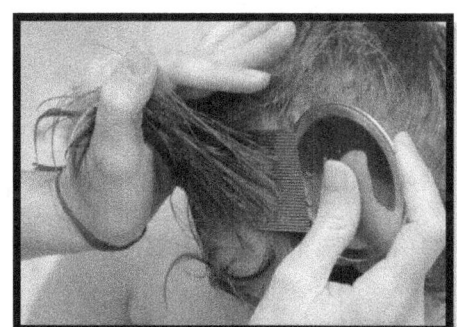

- **Burn them up.** Dry your hair with an electric hair dryer, combing it out with only 'clean' combs and brushes. Lice can't take the heat over 110F.

- **Smother them with Coconut or Olive oil.** Melt Coconut oil/Olive oil. Apply to scalp and hair liberally. Massage well into scalp down to the length of your hair. Wrap hair in a plastic cap and wear for at least a couple of hours…use shampoo that has tea tree oil in it, making sure to massage shampoo into scalp *without* scratching the scalp- and working through the hair. Rinse well with hottest water temperate you can stand.
Comb hair through with nit comb to remove all dead louse and eggs.

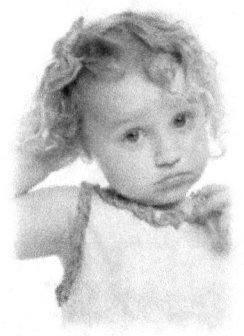

How to Prevent Lice and Nits

To prevent lice and nits from spreading, make sure that each person in the household has their own comb or brush. If one of you gets lice, there is a good chance that the others will not if they are not sharing combs or brushes. Your child must learn that they *must not* share a comb or brush at school or in the neighborhood with others.

Your child must also be taught that they can never wear anyone else's jackets, sweaters, barrettes, hats, helmets, etc., and that no one else may wear their things. If someone at school puts your child's hat on, your child must know to not put the hat on but instead bring it home for washing or bagging. Hats, sweaters and jackets must be kept isolated at school when your child is not wearing them, especially if there is an outbreak.

These items should go into a zipped up backpack or deep into their own "cubby." If all of the coats in the classroom are touching each other while hanging on a rack or hangers, lice could be marching from one to the next. It is a game of Russian roulette as to who would be the next child to bring the lice home - if not all of the children.

Keep your child out of the sandbox - or at least keep your child's hair out of the sand (and the sand out of your child's hair). If a child with lice puts his head in the sand, some lice could stay in the sand. Lice can stay alive for 24 hours or so, which is time enough to infect lots of heads when kids pour sand over each other. We have found that the kids who are always playing in the sand are also the first ones to be sent home with lice in every outbreak.

One of the best things to use to prevent lice is the right shampoo. Coconut oil and olive oil contain fatty acids that break down the bodies (exoskeletons) of the lice and kill them.

PART 2

WHAT CAUSES DANDRUFF?

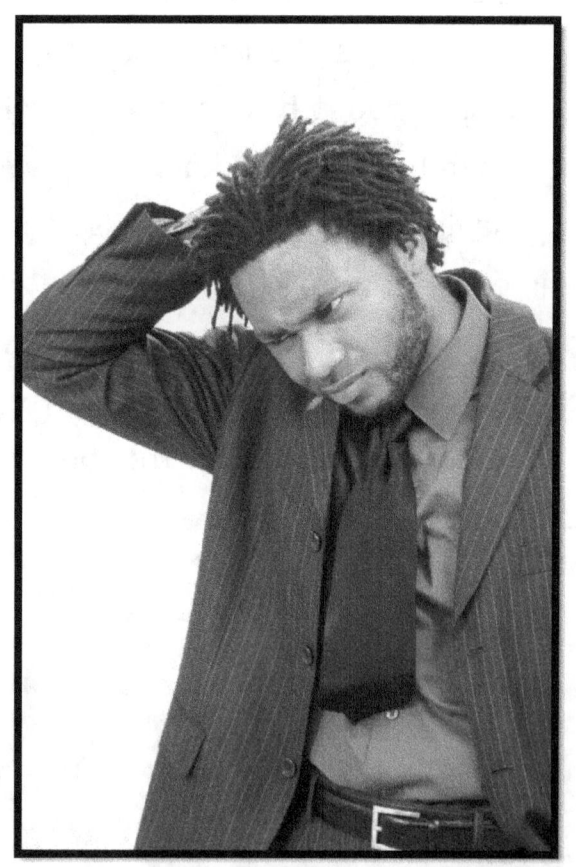

What causes Dandruff?

Although the problem of dandruff is probably one that has affected mankind almost since the dawn of time, it is nevertheless a problem that is not completely and fully understood as yet.

Hence it is difficult if not impossible to give a complete definition of what causes dandruff. On the other hand, there are many factors that appear to be implicated in causing the condition, some of which are internal, others that are directly related to the scalp itself.

Firstly, there are suggestions that part of the reason that some people suffer dandruff could be genetic. Part of the reason for believing this is that dandruff generally starts to appear after puberty, and is also far more common in men than it is in women. Another oddity about dandruff is that it appears to be more common in people who suffer from certain diseases, such as Parkinson's disease, which researchers suggest might also have some genetic causes as well.

Some 25 years ago, dermatologists began to suspect that one of the major causes of dandruff is naturally occurring yeast that everyone carries on their skin known as *Malassezia yeast*.

Malassezia and Dandruff - what is the correlation?

There are ongoing studies about the causes of dandruff in relation to the Malassezia yeast. A few different species of the yeast have been discovered. It was first suggested that the Malassezia furfur (M. furfur) fungus was the main cause. However, scientists have found that the scalp condition affecting more than 50% of Caucasians and 80% of people of African descent is caused by the lipid waste of two other Malassezia species, (M. restricta) and (M. globosa).

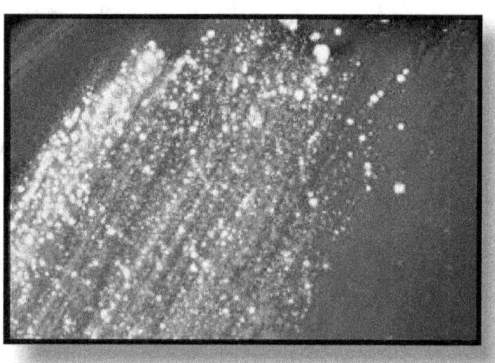

(Malassezia Restricta species)

**In a research study conducted by Thomas Dawson, Jr., Ph.D., and senior scientist in beauty care technology for P&G, titled, "Fast, Non-invasive Method for Molecular Detection and Speciation of Malassezia on Human Skin, and Application to Dandruff Microbiology," scalp samples from 70 people with dandruff showed the presence of Malassezia species. But in these cases, M. restricta was present in 70 percent and M. globosa in 45 percent. M. furfur was not detected in any of the samples.

Malassezia is a lipophilic fungal genus, members of which are part of the normal human scalp flora. M. restricta and M. globosa feed on lipids secreted from the hair follicles. The partially digested lipids that linger on the skin cause the familiar irritation of the scalp that leads to dandruff.

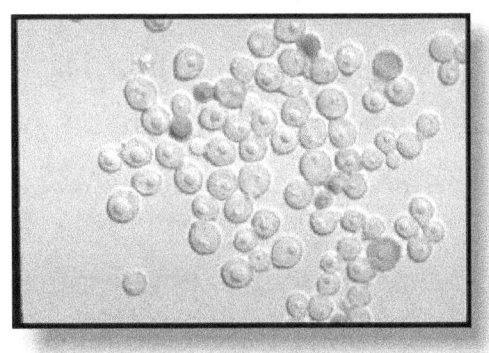

(Malassezia Globosa species)

"We have been studying dandruff and other scalp conditions for many years, concentrating on the specific organism that causes the disorder," said Dr. Dawson. "We expect these data will provide insight into the development of new approaches to dandruff treatment."

"These new data on the real cause of dandruff are a major step forward in understanding dandruff that will be important to the dermatology community," said Boni E. Elewski, MD, Professor of Dermatology at the University of Alabama, Birmingham, and internationally-recognized authority on cutaneous fungal infections and dandruff. "This research will allow development of more effective anti-dandruff treatments that will not only treat the condition, but may also help prevent it from occurring."

Dr. Dawson's findings also apply to Seborrheic dermatitis, a severe form of dandruff that affects up to 10 percent of Caucasians and leads to heavy flaking, severe itchiness, redness and inflammation. Earlier work by this team of P&G scientists has shown that excess lipids are correlated to dandruff and Seborrheic dermatitis, and this study showed that reducing the amount of sebum by more frequent washing improved the clinical signs of Seborrheic dermatitis. This also lends support to the theory that sebum has a positive effect on the growth of fungus. ***reference resource: hairlosshelp.com*

Nowadays, it is generally agreed that it is a combination of these particular species of yeast and the sebum secreted by the sebaceous glands in the hair upon which these particular yeasts feeds, that is the primary cause of dandruff in an individual who is already genetically predisposed to suffering from the condition.

When the Malassezia yeast feeds on the natural grease (sebum) produced by the human skin, it generates oleic acid which then penetrates the stratum cornea (the outermost layer of the skin) which causes irregularities in the way the skin cells divide, accelerating the growth of new cells by doing so.

As earlier suggested, it is this increased turnover or rapid production of skin cells that causes dandruff, and by removing Malassezia yeast from the skin, it should help to reduce or remove the dandruff problem.

Five Dandruff Facts

#1   Does dry skin cause dandruff?

It is a very common belief that dry skin and dandruff go together, but in fact, nothing could be further from the truth. As suggested in the previous chapter, without sebum, the Malassezia yeast has nothing to feed on and therefore the whole 'chain' of dandruff production is irrevocably broken without oily skin.

#2   Is Dandruff a result of poor hygiene?

It is unlikely that poor hygiene has anything to do with causing dandruff despite the fact that the probable main cause of the condition is yeast (Malassezia yeast) on the skin which feeds on the oil (sebum) secreted by the sebaceous glands.

However, it appears that people who suffer dandruff do not necessarily have more yeast on their skin, although they may at certain times of their life (i.e. around puberty) produce more natural oil. In fact, rather than having more yeast on their skin, it is likely that people who suffer from dandruff simply are more sensitive to the yeast.

#3   Sunlight and Headgear: Problem or Solution?

It is probably true that exposing your head to the sunlight may inhibit the growth of Malassezia yeast which like all other yeasts thrives in darker, damp conditions.

Think about the kind of places where you would expect fungi (yeast is a fungus) like mushrooms to grow, and you will quickly have a fairly accurate picture of the kind of conditions in which Malassezia yeast is happiest. And I have no doubt that the picture in your mind is not one of mushrooms shooting up in bright, warm sunlight!

It is for this reason that many people suspect (perhaps correctly) that wearing a hat or a bonnet might create an ideal environment for dandruff to develop, because enclosing your head in this way could create an environment that is far more likely for Malassezia yeast to thrive in.

For this reason, if you are a dandruff sufferer, one of the first things that you can do is to expose your head to the sunlight as often as you possibly can. In the same vein, you should avoid wearing headgear whenever possible as well.

Many sufferers find that their dandruff is seasonal, being considerably worse in the cold and damp of the fall (autumn) and winter than it is in spring and summer.

Of course, if you live in a place where sunlight is generally at a premium, there is perhaps not a great deal you can do, but you should nonetheless be aware that exposing your head to the sun is one way of naturally combating dandruff.

#4   Can you contract dandruff from a dirty hairbrush?

Although it may not be particularly pleasant to use someone else's hair brush or comb if they are a dandruff sufferer, it is not true that you can develop dandruff yourself from doing so. Unlike head lice (as an example), dandruff cannot be passed from one person to another in any way as it is entirely non-contagious, so sharing a brush or borrowing someone else's hat is not going to increase the possibility of you developing a dandruff problem.

#5   Stress and your diet: How are they connected?

There is evidence that stress can play a part in causing dandruff or in making a pre-existing dandruff problem worse. Why this should be the case is not particularly clear, although it may be that your body speeds up the skin cell production process at times of stress and anxiety when it is more excited.

There may also be a connection with the fact that stress and anxiety might prompt quicker sebum production as it is natural to sweat more at times when anxiety or stress is greater.

In a similar manner, if your diet contains too much sugar, fat, or starch, this could exacerbate your dandruff problem, as can a diet that is generally low in healthy nutrition.

It is sometimes suggested that a dandruff sufferer should avoid eating hot spicy food (which causes sweating in many people) and that alcohol should also be avoided as it is believed that the toxic nature of alcohol in the body might aggravate the problem.

PART 3

How to Combat Dandruff –

Putting it all Together

and

Taking Control

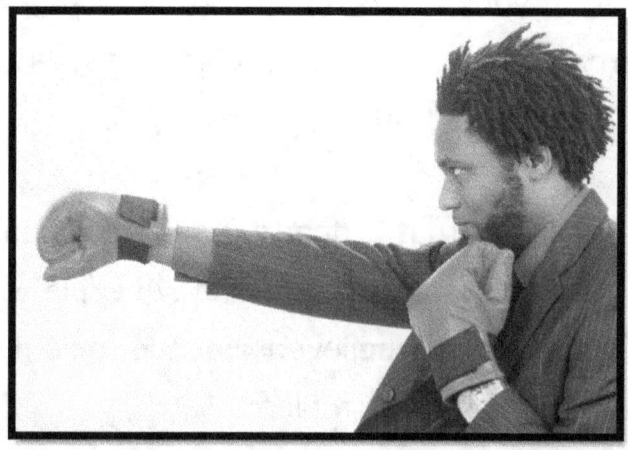

How to Combat Dandruff – Putting it all Together and Taking Control

Perhaps one more irritating factor for people who suffer dandruff is

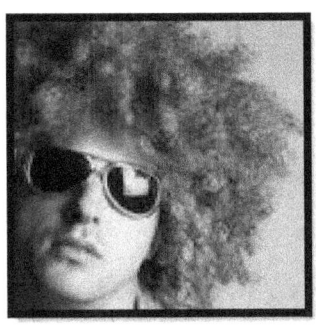

that it always seems as if the treatments that work superbly well for other people do not work at all for you.

Whether you are looking at chemical-based shampoos as highlighted in the previous chapter or whether you are considering natural dandruff treatments, the same always seems to apply.

You know someone who uses 'Brand X' shampoo or 'natural treatment Y', and it has got rid of their dandruff almost completely, and yet it does not seem to touch your condition at all.

This is a simple but extremely unfortunate result of the fact that every one of us is different, and we all react to different substances in a different way. In practical terms, what this means is that if you have dandruff, it is a matter of trial and error, testing various different ideas and solutions until you find something that works.

However, it is important that whenever you try different solutions for your dandruff problem, you should start with those that are the least likely to cause you adverse side-effects.

This almost inevitably means trying natural solutions before moving on to those based on chemicals if the natural solutions do not work. As I have already suggested, although most chemical-based shampoos do not carry significant risk of side-effects, there is nevertheless a degree of risk involved in using them.

And as you will discover in **Part 4- Natural Dandruff Treatments – recipes, herbs and other concoctions**, controlling your dandruff problem is not simply a matter of applying different substances to your scalp until you find one that works (although you will of course do so), the first thing that you should do to try to bring your dandruff problem under control is to consider your current lifestyle to assess whether there are any changes that you can make that could help to reduce your dandruff.

For example, in the next sections to follow, you will discover why many experts believe that stress and anxiety plays an active role in determining how bad (or how well controlled) your dandruff problem is.

Consequently, if you can reduce the level or degree of stress in your life, it stands to reason that this will represent a significant lifestyle improvement. This improvement should in turn make it easier to control your dandruff, which in itself will probably further reduce your stress and anxiety (it's a pleasant circle as opposed to a vicious one!).

Let us therefore consider some changes that you can make or regimens that you can introduce into your life which will help to reduce the adverse factors or conditions in your current lifestyle that can aggravate your dandruff problem.

Food: You Really Are What You Eat!

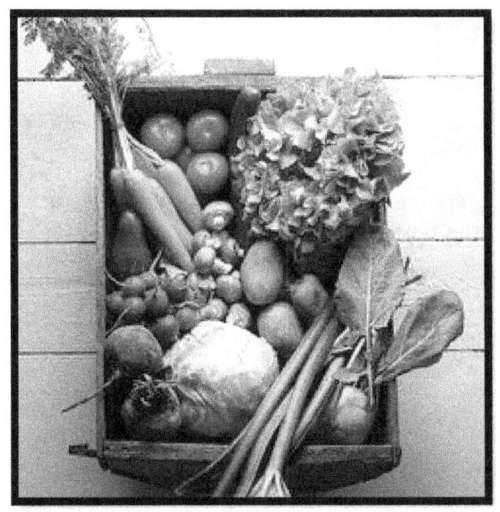

I know that it is a cliché, but from the day you were born, every centimeter that you have added to your frame has been put there as a direct result of the food you eat and the beverages you drink. It is therefore absolutely, 100% true that you are what you eat (and drink of course).

From this, it naturally follows that everything you eat and drink has a profound effect on your general well-being, health and overall life. Consequently, if you suffer from a problem like dandruff, while you might be genetically predisposed to it, it does not necessarily mean that you have to accept it without attempting to fight back.

Part of this fighting back process has got to be reassessing what you currently eat and drink every day to see whether there are improvements you can make which might help to control your dandruff, and offer a better quality of life- period.

As suggested previously, you should try to avoid eating a diet that is too rich and too spicy, because not only is there a chance that spicy foods might increase your bodily secretions, it is also a fact that some spices irritate the average human metabolism. When your body is irritated, it naturally tries to counteract this irritation by fighting back which in turn can lead to internal imbalances.

Internal imbalances will often manifest themselves in sickness, and are susceptible to infections and other external indications of imbalance, one of which could well be worsened dandruff.

Because there are other foodstuffs that you should reduce (or completely cut from your diet), your intake of them is believed to have a direct effect on the production of sebum which feeds the yeast that leads to dandruff.

For example, cutting down on the saturated fats of the kind that are contained in red meat such as beef while also reducing your intake of trans-fatty acids that are often found in margarine could help to reduce your susceptibility to dandruff, because both of these forms of fat are believed to encourage increased sebum production.

Whether you are a dandruff sufferer or not, it is common knowledge that a diet rich in colorful fruits and vegetables is always good for you, but what might not be that well known is that it is a particularly good idea for someone with dandruff to eat a vegetable and fruit rich diet. Many of these foods are rich in minerals and B vitamins and it is generally accepted that a deficiency of both of these nutrients can aggravate a dandruff problem.

Hence, you should include a good portion of leafy green vegetables, potatoes, bananas, red chili peppers and lentils in your diet as all of these are a rich source of different minerals and vitamin B variants. The B vitamins help to counteract the inefficient metabolism of fatty acids and carbohydrates which is in turn believed to contribute to the incidence of dandruff, so increasing the level of these vitamins in your diet is a significant step towards freeing yourself of the misery of dandruff.

If you do not consume milk (or soymilk; more on this later), as part of your everyday diet, you should, because it contains every vitamin that mammals need for good health. The fat soluble vitamins such as vitamin A, K, D, and E, are all contained in the milk fat, so if you drink non-fat or reduced fat milk, you will not take in much of any of these vitamins.

On the other hand, the B group vitamins are found in the aqueous (water based) part of the milk, so even if you drink reduced fat milk, you will still get a significant amount of B vitamins. Incidentally, fluid milk in the USA is often supplemented with vitamin D, while in other countries, different vitamin supplements are added to fluid milk, such as vitamin A.

It is also believed that vitamin D3 has many benefits, particularly for your skin. Unfortunately, the human body does not generate vitamin D without some outside assistance although each and every one of us needs vitamin D in order to maintain good health. However, it is generated primarily by the skin due to the effects of sunlight in combination with certain foodstuffs such as milk, cheese, butter, cereals and fatty fish.

Of course, many of us see very little of the sun, perhaps because we live in a part of the world where there is not a great deal of sunshine for a significant proportion of the year, or perhaps because the majority of people work in an indoor environment. It is for these reasons that vitamin D deficiency is most commonly seen in people who live in the northern regions at higher latitudes who see less of the sun than people that live close to the equator.

Furthermore, even for people who live in sunnier climates, their concern over the possibility of contracting skin cancer leads many to use sunscreen every time they venture outdoors. While taking such precautions is obviously sensible in some ways, it does unfortunately mean that perhaps as much as 95% of the body's ability to generate vitamin D is cancelled out by the application of sunscreen.

Recent studies have indicated that many patients who are suffering from a wide variety of inflammatory conditions were vitamin D deficient. The connection between vitamin D and inflammatory conditions (of which dandruff is one example) was further emphasized by the fact that

the condition of many of these patients improved once additional vitamin D was added to their diet.

There are various different forms in which vitamin D can be taken, but it is generally agreed that vitamin D3, the form that is typically found in fish oil or other oily fish related products is the most beneficial because it appears to be the form from which vitamin D can be absorbed most efficiently.

Some nutritionists suggest that increasing the amount of gamma-linolenic acid (GLA) in your diet can also assist anyone with a dandruff problem to minimize the size of that problem.

It is believed that increasing the amount of GLA in your diet will help to improve the general condition of your skin and hair, so it is probably worth adding a rich source of GLA such as blackcurrant or evening primrose oil to your diet to see what difference this makes.

So the question is: Can water cure dandruff?

I've discovered an article dated back a couple years, written by Jointer West. Jointer is a Yahoo contributor. I'm sharing it here, because I think it is relevant to this question: *Can water cure dandruff?*

How to Cure Dandruff Using Only Cool Water by Jointer West

I am a 28 year old male who has suffered from dandruff. As a child I was tortured by dandruff. It seemed like nobody at school liked a 'dirty' peer.
I do not use "Head and Shoulders". And I do not use any type of formulated shampoo. This is a natural and cheap method for curing dandruff.

Years and years ago my Ant tried to show me how to cure dandruff. I would not do it, because I was not comfortable someone with me in a bathroom. Especially if I am naked.

It is very simple, and easy to do. The only ingredient is water. The trick is using cold water, and not hot or warm.

The way I do it, is I take my hot or warm shower as normal. I clean myself with soap, and wash my hair with shampoo and conditioner.

Before I cut the water off, I turn down the hot side. I don't turn it all the way off, because the cold water is just too cold for me. I turn it down enough that the water is cool, and not warm.

I then just rinse off in the cool water. I find it very refreshing to rinse off in cool water after a shower. Rinsing my hair out, which is why I cool it down. It not only solves my dandruff problem, but it makes me feel cleaner.

Dandruff can be caused by coming out of a warm or hot shower, with the warm or hot water on your scalp. It has something to do with the temperature change.

When I step out with cool water on my scalp, I don't get the dandruff. I know there is a little bit of dandruff. But it's nothing like stepping out with warm water on my head.

Kids would make fun of me, and tell me it's snowing. But using the cold water method, there is no snow. I guess I made it to spring, and out of winter!

I don't think this can cure dandruff caused by a fungus, or other reasons like that for dandruff. But it cures mine, and it also prevents it.

When winter comes, I usually end up with dandruff. This is because of the cold water. It is torture to use the cold water in winter. I end up being weak, and step out with hot water on me. It gives me a bad case of dandruff. But when spring and summer are here, no dandruff.

Soymilk: What are the Benefits

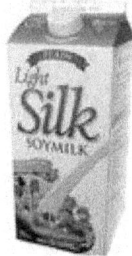 Soy milk is made from soybeans and is said to be good for our health. Soy milk is high in protein, and because it is made from beans, it also contains considerably more fiber than cow's milk. Soy milk is low in calories and doesn't include cholesterol. It is a good source of protein and vitamins, such as vitamin B1, B2, B6, and E. Soy milk is rich in minerals, such as magnesium.

Besides the extra protein and fiber, the biggest benefit in soy milk is the isoflavones. Sounds complex, but basically isoflavones are actually chemicals very similar to the hormone estrogen. Isoflavones are connected to a whole host of health issues, with the most prevalent being the *prevention* of many cancers, heart disease, osteoporosis and more.

Soy milk contains calcium, and essential fatty acids. While high in dietary fiber, soy milk is low in sodium and saturated fat. Soy protein helps men to grow and also nourish hair.

Soy milk is lactose-free, making it ideal for people suffering from lactose-intolerance. As an added bonus, soy milk is also free of casein, a protein found in cow's milk that causes many allergic reactions and gastrointestinal problems.

Soy milk can be a great alternative to cow's milk. If you don't have a soy allergy, try using soy milk in any recipe where cow's milk is used.

De-Stress and Wash Those Flakes Away

A degree of stress in your life is not always a bad thing. It can make you more alert and helps to build character and endurance. However, there are times when it all gets too much, and when that happens, one result can be a marked worsening in your dandruff.

Repetitive stress brings on chronic fatigue, meaning that your health and wellbeing can suffer in many ways; one, being a negative change that can be reflected in worsening dandruff. For instance, stress can lead to depression, a lack of energy, insomnia and hair loss as well as deteriorating dandruff, so it obviously makes sense to keep the stress in your life to a manageable level.

There are extremely simple but effective ways you can de-stress yourself. In order to get the maximum relaxation from what is for most people an immensely pleasurable experience, **here are a few things that you should make sure you do:**

1. **Take a nice warm bath every day**. When done right, it is one of the best ways of relaxing, one that far too few people really give serious credence to.

2. **Pay attention to the temperature of the water**. You have never heard anyone advise you to take a nice *cold* bath, right? That's because cold is not something that most of us would consider to be nice or conducive to being relaxed. Hot water of between 35 degrees (96°F) and 39 degrees Celsius (102°F) is ideal for relaxing the muscles, improving your circulation, soothing your nerves and giving your immune system a 'pep-up'.

3. **Think about the environment that you bathe in and how**

you can improve it to aid your efforts in relaxing completely. Mood music soft and gentle – can definitely help, possibly because as the experts point out, we all listened to the sound of our mother's heartbeat when we were in the womb and were relaxed by it. Hence, recreating a similar protective environment by using relaxing sounds or music can return us to that happier, more relaxed state.

The lighting in your bathroom can also have a big positive effect. Low lights almost always help you to relax more completely, this is because when it is darker, your body naturally reacts by increasing the secretion of a hormone called *melatonin*, which is produced by the pineal gland in your brain in response to the dimmer light. Melatonin makes you drowsy, which is why it is easier for most people to go to sleep at night when it is dark than it is during the daylight hours.

Aromatherapy is something that should become an integral part of your de-stressing bath time routine, irrespective of age or gender.

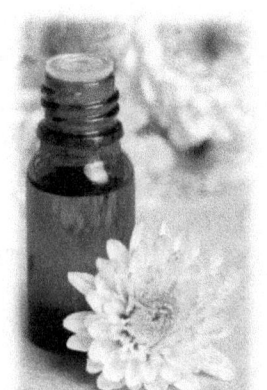 Using aromatic bath oils is a terrific way of relaxing, because not only does the heat from the water make it easier for the relaxing oil molecules to permeate your skin, it also releases those molecules into the air as well.

Unlike the other senses, something that you smell has direct access to your brain via your olfactory receptors, hence it is known that aromatic oils that you inhale can have a direct effect on your hormones, your brain chemistry and stress levels.

Tests have indicated that there are certain essential oils that are particularly good for relieving stress, such as lavender oil or chamomile. Of the group of around 40 such oils and herbs that can play a significant role in ensuring that you are as relaxed as possible, others are dandelion, burdock root, peppermint, rosemary and juniper.

If at all possible, you should plan to take a relaxing hot bath in an ideal environment using aromatic oils at least once a day. By having and sticking to a 'planned out in advance' strategy in this way, it should be relatively easy to make sure that you always have essential oils that you need in the house.

Relaxing Concoctions - Use What You Have

However, there may be times when oils are not available, so you might need to *manufacture* something that can act as an effective aromatic-oils stand-in from common household substances.

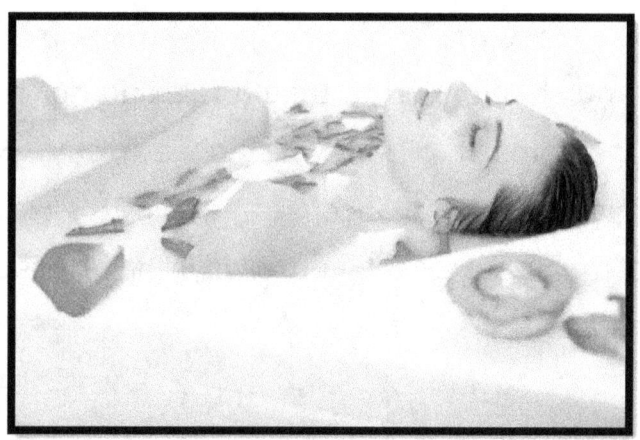

Here are a few suggestions:

1. **Herbal Teabags**- If you have herbal teabags available, drop a couple of them in your bath water before immersing yourself. Yes, the water may turn a slightly strange color, but it is not going to stain you forever, and the upside benefits will far outweigh any potential downside.

2. **Baby Oil**- mix a ¼ cup of baby oil with one tablespoonful of vanilla extract, and use the mixture in the bath.

3. **Slices of citrus fruits**- orange, lemons and grapefruit works extremely well, particularly because grapefruit releases encephalin into the air which are natural painkillers.

4. **Mix ½ cup of honey** together with two cups of cheap red wine (even older, oxidized wine is fine) and use this mixture in your bath water.

Any of these mixtures will help to create the relaxing bath time atmosphere that you need to remove harmful stress from your life. If by taking a bath every day in this way you can significantly reduce the anxiety and stress that you feel, it will help to boost your general well-being, which in turn represents a significant step to reducing your dandruff problem.

Relax Your Mind and Free Your Soul - Yoga, Meditation and Breathing to Combat Stress

It is generally accepted that practicing yoga, learning to meditate and how to breathe properly will all help to reduce the stress that you might feel on a day-to-day basis.

The best part about learning any of these practices is that there is so much information available on the net that can help you to get started. These resources are invaluable, because they allow you to have a go at yoga, meditation and learning to breathe properly before deciding whether it is for you.

The advantages of being able to learn about and to try these practices in the comfort of your own home should be relatively easy to appreciate. Not only can you learn at your own speed without having to leave home, you do not need to enroll in a class (and spend money) only to find that yoga or whatever it is, does not suit your lifestyle or preferences.

Obviously, yoga or meditation is not for everyone, but because these practices are widely accepted to *teach* people who are adept at them how to relax and therefore minimize stress, each of them is worth investigating further and trying.

For instance, by looking at sites for *learning yoga*, you can learn plenty about the history of yoga, what it can do for you and how you can get started at home. Search Google for 'yoga', and you will find plenty more similar resources that can teach you everything you could ever need to know about yoga and its benefits.

Similarly, try a Google search for *meditation* or *learning meditation* and *breathing* or *deep breathing* to find all of the information and resources that you could need in order to get you started.

Once again, reducing your everyday stress levels will improve your dandruff, and all of these practices will help to reduce stress.

While you might not have ever considered yoga, meditation or learning to breathe properly as practices that could help to combat your dandruff problem, they almost certainly can and will, so they're all worth trying.

Four Therapeutic Ways to Minimize Dandruff

#1   Aromatherapy

In addition to using aromatherapy at bath time as highlighted in the previous chapter, a leading herbalist Jeanne Rose (Director of the Institute of Aromatic Studies) suggests a more direct use of aromatic oils as a way of combating dandruff. Her suggestion is that after washing your hair, you should let your hair dry completely before massaging a few drops each of lemon and rosemary oils into your scalp.

Mix the two oils together and squeeze small drops in your scalp and massage thoroughly.

These oils have natural antifungal characteristics, meaning that they will fight to keep the amount of yeast on your scalp to a minimum.

#2   Ayurveda

It is suggested by leading expert, David Frawley, that dandruff is a condition caused by poor or blocked circulation. He has suggested a couple of possible solutions to this problem.

The first option is to massage sesame oil into your scalp for 5 or 10 minutes once or twice a week immediately before taking your evening shower. After massaging the oil in, allow it to 'sit' for a few minutes before washing it out in the shower.

Alternatively, Dr. Frawley also suggests that fenugreek is a recognized treatment for dandruff in Ayurveda medicine. It is also a spice that is widely used in Asian cooking, so you can either add it to your own home cooking or you can take it as a powder mixed with honey.

#3 Homeopathy

According to one of the UK's leading medically qualified homeopaths, Dr. Andrew Lockie, there are quite a few homeopathic treatments that can be very effective for combating dandruff.

According to Dr. Lockie, you should try using sulphur if you find yourself persistently scratching your head at night or if your scalp burns and you have thick, heavy dandruff. Try massaging sulphur into your scalp three or four times a week for a period of two weeks, and you should find that your dandruff eases considerably.

On the other hand, he suggests that sepia will soothe your scalp if it is greasy, moist and sensitive to the touch around the roots.

However, when you are massaging these soothing substances into your scalp (or any other substances for that matter), do take care that you do not massage it into your skull too vigorously. Studies have indicated that if you are too vigorous and energetic, you will damage your hair around the roots which can speed up your natural hair loss process.

Consequently, you should try to avoid significant amounts of contact between your fingernails and your scalp, particularly around the roots, because it is your nails that are likely to cause most damage, and damage makes your hair fall out much more quickly.

A third option that is suggested by Dr. Lockie is to use oleander if you feel that the palpable irritation from your dandruff is worsened by heat, or if you feel as if your head is covered in insect bites.

All three substances suggested by Dr. Lockie can be obtained at health food stores online and offline and possibly some pharmacies as well.

According to some research, adding flaxseed oil to your diet can help to significantly reduce the amount of oil that your skin secretes, and as we have already seen, it is the sebum that your skin secretes that provides the Malassezia yeast with something to feed and thrive on.

It is suggested that two or three teaspoonfuls of flaxseed oil every day (or the equivalent amount in capsules) will significantly reduce the amount of sebum you secrete, thereby reducing the 'yeast food' on your scalp which should in turn reduce your dandruff.

#4 Enema

An Enema is a method to flush waste out of the colon. It's not such a bad idea when you consider that the average person may have up to 10 pounds or more of non-eliminated waste in the large intestine.

Simply put, an enema cleans up the colon and induces bowel movements, leaving you feeling cleaner, lighter and healthier almost immediately.

The main job of the colon is to absorb water and nutrients from food and remove waste and toxins. Over the years the colon walls can become encrusted with non-eliminated waste, making it sluggish and inefficient. When that happens, you might experience some of the following symptoms:

- Allergies
- Loss of Appetite
- Irritability
- Depression
- Swelling
- Weight Problems
- Fatigue
- Headache
- Inability to Concentrate
- Indigestion
- Stomach Pains

Most people greet the notion of a home enema with a wince and a snicker. Knowing the benefits of an enema can change that wince into a whisper of relief.

Clean water is the key ingredient to a home enema. Add herbs, probiotics or minerals for an effective way to soothe and cleanse the colon.

If you've read the Body Ecology Diet you know that good health begins right in the gut. Eating a natural, wholesome diet with fermented foods, drinking clean water, exercising, getting plenty of rest, and breathing fresh air is essential for proper digestion, vibrant health and well-being.

But all of your efforts toward a healthy diet and lifestyle could go right down the drain if you're not eliminating properly!

When waste material travels too slowly through the intestines or you become constipated and they literally jam up, putrefaction and toxins occur. Constipation is damaging to every cell and to every organ in our body not just to our intestines. Our bodies are designed to absorb whatever is in the digestive tract... good or bad.

So in other words, if you begin your meal with healthy foods, and if you chew and digest them well, your body will absorb truly valuable nutrients. But if you leave putrefying, toxic waste in your system, your body will absorb that too. That's the point where autointoxication or self-poisoning occurs.

Enemas are not a new fad or something that's only performed by those obsessed with their health. It wasn't that long ago that enema's were routinely prescribed by doctors as part of a normal cure for illness.

Today the medical community has somehow disconnected itself with the benefits of enemas, and so it is up to us individually to take back our health and start adding this powerful tradition back into our lifestyle to maintain good health.

Let's take a look at what you could see disappear with regular enemas:

- Constipation
- Candida Yeast Infections (psoriasis etc.)

- Backache

- Fatigue

- Bloating

- Indigestion

- Weight Issues

- Skin Conditions (dandruff, ringworm, psoriasis, Seborrheic dermatitis etc.)

- Headaches

- Hemorrhoids

- Sinus Congestion

- Flatulence

- Loss of Concentration

- Unpleasant Breath

If you experience any of those conditions, perhaps you should consider an Enema.

Following are the steps to giving yourself an enema-- taken from the *TummyTemple.com*. I personally use the same method as explained below.

How To Give Yourself An Enema

An enema is a great way to stimulate a bowel movement. It will not cleanse the entire intestine nor will it condition the muscle. However, it can bring instant relief when you are "in a bind".

Equipment Needed

• An enema bag. You can obtain this in any pharmacy.

• K-Y Jelly or any edible oil. This is used to make insertion of the rectal tube easier and more comfortable.

• Something to hang the bag if self-administered. The enema bag should be suspended no more than 18-24 inches above the level of the rectum.

• A good location: the best place to give yourself an enema is on the bed or in the bathroom either lying on a rug or in the bathtub.

• A pad or heavy bath towel to be placed underneath the buttocks during the enema.

• A healthy source of water. Your colon will be absorbing this water into your body. Use the same water you would drink, preferably filtered or spring water.

Procedure

For best results, and your own comfort, the enema should be taken while lying down. If you will be giving the enema to yourself the first thing you should do is set up the area for the procedure. Make sure the hook is suspended at the proper height (18-24 inches above the rectum). Then place a pad or bath towel where you will be lying down. Slide the shutoff clamp to a point on the tubing where you will be able to easily reach it while in position.

Check this out ahead of time by hanging the empty bag and assuming the position, just to be sure. Prepare the solution. The water temperature should be slightly above body temperature, between 98 and 105 degrees F at time of use. You may need to heat water on the stove but BE SURE NOT TO USE HOT water that could hurt you, cool it down if necessary till it's comfortable to the touch.

Fill the enema bag 90% full with the water. Lubricate the rectal nozzle with K-Y jelly or oil. Open the shutoff for a moment and allow enough solution to flow to expel the air from the enema tubing. This helps to reduce cramping. Lubricate your anal area with a generous amount of K-Y Jelly or oil. Work your index finger up into the rectum lubricating the entire interior area where you can reach.

Hang the enema bag on the hook. Lie down in position. On the bed this should be on the left side with the left leg straight and the right knee flexed (Sim's position). Your left arm should be behind your back and if the shutoff is properly positioned you will be able to control it with your left hand. Your right hand will comfortably rest under your pillow.

On the bathroom floor or in the tub, lie on your back with both legs drawn up, knees bent. Make sure you can easily reach the shutoff valve. Put a pillow under your head.

If someone else is giving you the enema you may find it more comfortable to assume the knee-chest position. To accomplish this, get on your hands and knees and then put one or two pillows underneath your chest, and lean forward on them.

Turn your face sideways and rest it on another pillow, and snuggle both arms underneath. This particular position is an especially comfortable one to have an enema during pregnancy, but if you attempt it on your own the rectal tube tends to slip out and it is difficult to work the shutoff. If you do this on the bathroom floor rather than the bed, make sure your knees are cushioned by a pillow or a pad, or the pressure on them might cause knee damage.

Gently insert the rectal tube 3 to 4 inches into the rectum. Rotate or twist the tube back and forth to make for easier insertion. Open the shutoff valve and allow the solution to flow.

At the first indication of discomfort stop and wait a few moments. Then release the shutoff and allow the enema to resume. Feel free to interrupt the flow as frequently as is necessary to assist in minimizing the discomfort.

Taking slow deep breaths will help, and if you feel cramping at any point "pant like a dog" with shallow quick breathing. As the enema progresses a feeling of fullness will develop. This is normal, and discomfort can be minimized by insuring that not too much solution is introduced too quickly. Take your time.

When the bag is empty clamp off the shutoff and slowly remove the rectal tube. Remain in position and retain the solution for a while. For a maintenance enema a few minutes are sufficient, but if you are constipated try to hold it in for 5 to 15 minutes.

Go to the toilet and expel the enema. An enema seldom comes out in a single movement so stay near the toilet for one half to one hour. After evacuating, most people find it comfortable to lie on the bed in a prone position to rest for a while.

Clean the equipment thoroughly and hang it all up to dry. An enema bag takes several days to thoroughly dry out, and should never be put away while even slightly wet.

Tips For Minimizing Discomfort

There are three primary reasons that cause an enema to be a more uncomfortable procedure than it has to be:

• Wrong position: Use the positions suggested here and don't give yourself and enema while seated on a toilet.

• Wrong temperature: An enema solution too cool can cause excessive cramping. If it is too hot it can damage the delicate mucosa lining the bowel. Body temperature or slightly above (98-105F) is just right.

• Too much pressure: If the bag or can is suspended too high, excessive pressure can cause severe discomfort. The bag should be just high enough to allow the solution to barely flow

Tips For Maximizing Results

• Use a sufficient volume of solution

• Retain the solution for 5 to 15 minutes.

• Retaining the enema for a while before expelling it can significantly contribute to good results.

Vitamins and Minerals for a Healthy Scalp

Earlier in this book, I highlighted the importance of eating a healthy

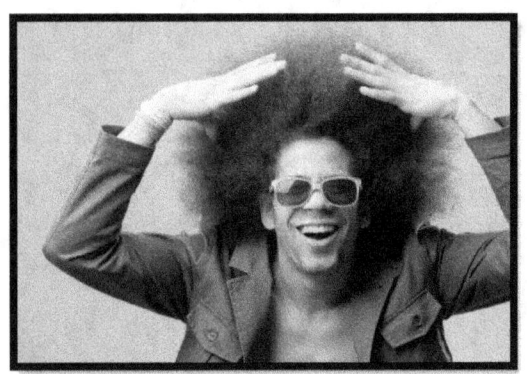

balanced diet in your efforts to reduce or get rid of your dandruff problem.

Unfortunately however, for many people, eating a healthy balanced diet every day is extremely difficult or impossible, primarily because with work and the day-to-day demands of living, it is simply too difficult to eat a healthy balanced meal at every meal time.

It is also true that in the modern world, many of the foods that we eat do not contain the vitamins and minerals that they should because far too often, those vitamins and minerals have been removed in the process of getting that food from its origin to your table.

For instance, unless you buy only organic vegetables, many of the vegetables that you are eating will have been grown in soil which is lacking in the minerals that form a very important part of a healthy diet. This is a natural side-effect of the fact that the demands on farming are increasingly heavy, meaning that the farmers who are responsible for growing the vegetables that you eat are forced into growing vegetables in soil of increasingly poor quality.

Taking these different factors into consideration, it becomes evident that there are many who will not get the necessary vitamins and nutrients through their food, whether they are conscious of this or not.

Consequently, dandruff sufferers who are not eating a healthy balanced diet are aggravating the severity of their problem internally.

For this situation to be turned around, supplementation of your diet with vitamins and minerals is therefore necessary.

The vitamins and minerals that you need to add to your diet if you suffer from dandruff are as follows, with an indication of what each of these vitamins and minerals will do for you:

- Vitamin B12 is believed to increase energy levels at the root level of your hair

- Vitamins B3, B5 and B6 stimulate healthy hair growth and stimulate the scalp

- Vitamin C encourages growth and improves circulation throughout the body, including on the scalp

- Vitamin D helps to control inflammatory conditions such as dandruff and psoriasis

- Iron helps to maintain the basic health of your hair, particularly the roots

- Zinc is an antibacterial that can help to fight the yeast on your scalp

- Folic acid helps to minimize hair loss

All of these nutrients stimulate the blood supply to your scalp, which in turn helps the top of your head to stay healthier. In effect, by making sure that all of these vitamins and nutrients are included either in your diet or in supplements, you are ensuring that you are dealing with your dandruff problem from the "root" (in more ways than one).

You are combating the problem internally by providing what your body needs to fight your problem completely naturally, so the importance of supplementing the kind of poor diet that many of us simply have to live with cannot be underestimated.

Commercial Anti-Dandruff Shampoo-- Analyzed

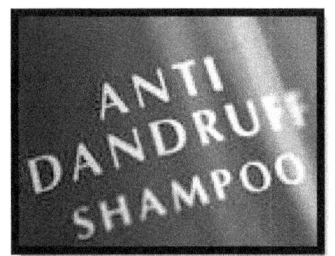

Perhaps not surprisingly, the number one objective of anyone who suffers from dandruff will almost inevitably be to do whatever is necessary to bring their condition under control. In fact, some of my clients who have suffered from dandruff, have tried almost every possible solution they have come across for the condition, including quite a few that (in truth) sounded extremely unlikely to work, if not a bit crazy!

Amongst the solutions that I would guess almost every dandruff sufferer has tried or will try are medicated shampoos; shampoos which include chemicals which are supposed to control dandruff.

There are many different anti-dandruff control shampoos on the market today, many of which can be bought over the counter in pharmacies or from drug stores. The active ingredients of these shampoos varies from one brand to another, with some being based on relatively natural substances while others are chemical based.

Before considering how you can treat your dandruff problem using commercial anti-dandruff shampoo brands, doesn't it make sense to research these shampoos first in order to establish whether there are any possible adverse side-effects?

In the majority of cases, the idea of including chemicals in an anti-dandruff shampoo is that the chemicals used are antimicrobial or antifungal so that they reduce or prevent dandruff by inhibiting the growth of the necessary yeast that is a root cause of dandruff.

There are several different chemicals used in the different brands, with the most common being selenium sulfide, pyrithione zinc and ketoconazole.

For the majority of people, because these chemicals are contained in relatively small amounts in medicated shampoos, the risk of adverse side-effects is fairly limited. However, this does not mean that there is no risk in using the shampoos, because every individual is different and therefore the susceptibility to unpleasant side-effects of any individual person using such a shampoo is relatively unknown.

For example, in the case of shampoos based on selenium sulfide, it is known that this particular chemical can exaggerate pre-existing dry or oily skin, and skin irritation is quite common. In more extreme cases, selenium sulfide can accelerate natural hair loss, which it is to be assumed is not the primary intention of anyone who is using a medicated shampoo to get rid of their dandruff!

Shampoos that contain pyrithione zinc are generally safe for most people, but some people do suffer allergic reactions to the chemical such as skin rashes, hives and lesions.

It should also be noted that several sources suggest that using pyrithione zinc based cleansing agent such as a shampoo over a prolonged period of time might increase the chance of adverse side-effects, so caution is necessary because it cannot be said with any certainty that pyrithione zinc is categorically safe. You should therefore be on the lookout for skin irritations or skin that does not heal as well as it did previously, and if either of these is encountered, you should report the fact to your medical attendant.

Shampoos that are based on ketoconazole are using a substance that is known to cause itching, nausea, vomiting, headache and abdominal pain, dizziness and fatigue. In extreme examples, it is believed that ketoconazole can even cause blood disorders and impotence so using a shampoo based on this particular chemical antifungal agent is something that you should do with extreme caution.

In tests, shampoos containing ketoconazole have been shown to be more effective than those that contain pyrithione zinc. On the other hand, it is also established that the possible side-effects of ketoconazole are considerably more unpleasant or dangerous than those of the zinc compound. In simple terms, ketoconazole is potentially more effective, but it is also potentially more dangerous as well.

The truth about using antifungal chemical based shampoos is that in the majority of cases, they are unlikely to do anyone significant harm, particularly on a short-term basis. This is relevant, because although dandruff is a chronic condition that can often be with you for a lifetime and (may be curable), it is also a condition that is seasonal.

Hence, you might find that while it is necessary during the colder, damper months to use a medicated shampoo containing one of the chemicals highlighted in this chapter, it may be unnecessary to use that shampoo all year round. This is something that will depend upon where you live and the severity of your condition, but it is nevertheless true that if you choose to use a chemical based medicated shampoo, you should try to avoid doing so on a permanent basis.

And of course, if any of the side-effects highlighted in this chapter become apparent, you should report the details about your condition to your medical attendant as soon as possible.

Dandruff Shampoo – A Non-Chemical Natural Approach

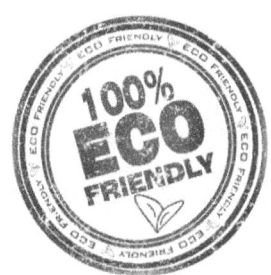 There are some anti-dandruff shampoos in the market today that are based on natural or relatively natural substances that you might want to consider using as an alternative to those that contain potentially damaging chemicals.

The two most effective natural ingredients in which a couple of commercially produced shampoos use are based on natural substances -*tea tree oil* and/or *coal tar*.

There are shampoos for dandruff on the market that have claims to work. However, many dandruff sufferers find that because of the chemical compounds that make up the product, the harsh detergents and chemicals perpetuate their problem.

Shampoos and conditioners that contain tea tree oil, peppermint or eucalyptus oil, lavender oil, and rosemary oil are really effective in relieving and soothing the scalp. Tea tree oil relieves dandruff and cradle cap. Shampoos and conditioners that contain tea tree oil are also great for use after a lice infestation (lice hate the smell so they stay away!) because it heals and soothes all of those little bites and sore skin from scratching.

What Is Tea Tree Oil?

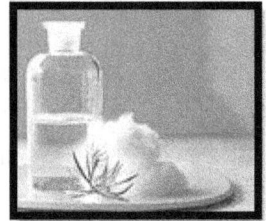 Tea tree oil is taken from the Melaleuca Alternifolia tree (botanical name) that is found on the north-east coast of New South Wales in Australia. It's a natural antibacterial, antiseptic, germicidal and fungicidal oil that has been used for hundreds of years as a medicinal treatment for a huge range of medical conditions by the native peoples of Australia.

Given all of these qualities possessed by tea tree oil, it is not surprising that it should be an effective additive to many leading brands of anti-dandruff shampoos. The natural antifungal qualities of tea tree oil will help to keep down the amount of yeast on your scalp, with most commercially produced tea tree oil based shampoos containing around 5% of the oil, which has been shown to be the most effective concentration in a commercially produced shampoo.

In fact, extensive research in Australia as reported in 2002 in the Journal of the American Academy of Dermatology indicated that a tea tree oil shampoo with 5% concentration of oil improved dandruff for 41% of people tested. From this statistic, there can be little doubt that tea tree oil shampoo is probably the most effective of the commercially produced shampoos based on natural substances for minimizing the worst effects of dandruff.

It is also effective for getting rid of head lice as well, so if it is lice that are causing what appeared to be a dandruff problem, this is an easy way to get rid of your unwanted guests.

There are no known adverse side-effects from using tea tree oil, although it is not a substance that you can ingest, so if you get tea tree oil shampoo in your mouth, you should immediately rinse it out with a plentiful supply of water.

Coal Tar Shampoo

Shampoo that is based on coal tar uses a substance that is produced as a byproduct of the carbonization of coal. Coal tar shampoo is often an effective treatment for dandruff, although because there is some concern that using coal tar in too great a concentration might possibly have some carcinogenic elements, you should ensure that any coal tar shampoo you use contains only a trace of coal tar.

My Recommendation

**Following, is my personal recommendation for a brand of shampoo that is amazingly effective, highly concentrated and excellent for scalp issues that have been discussed here in this book.

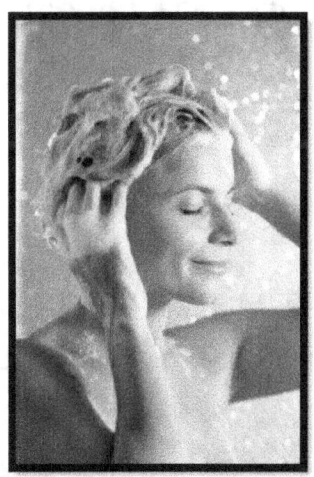

I highly recommend **Melaleuca Original Shampoo®**. It is your secret weapon against dry hair and itchy scalp. Here's why—
Melaleuca Alternifolia (tea tree oil) which is in the Melaleuca Original Shampoo®, has **six amazing properties** that makes it exceptional—

1. **Naturally Antiseptic**—Melaleuca oil helps stop topical bacteria so you have less possibilities of infection; paving the way for faster healing.

2. **Gently Soothes**—Melaleuca oil takes the 'ouch' out of minor cuts, burns and abrasions and bug bites. It calms dry itchy skin.

3. **Safely penetrates**—Melaleuca oil carries its healing benefits below the top skin layer, so you feel relief right where irritation begins.

4. **Beneficially Non-Caustic**—T36-C5® Melaleuca oil is mild on most skin types and T40-C3® Melaleuca oil is ideal for more sensitive skin.

5. **Effectively Solvent**—Melaleuca oil is a natural cleanser. As it kills bacteria, it also gently helps clean dirt and debris out of cuts and scrapes, jump starting the healing process.

6. **Pleasantly Aromatic**—Melaleuca oil has a natural, pleasing scent- never artificial or 'medicinal'.

For intense hair and scalp therapy, there's nothing like ***Melaleuca Original Shampoo®***. With a high concentration of pure T36-C5® Melaleuca oil (tea tree oil), shampoo penetrates deeply to wash away buildup and flakes, and helps to soothe dry, itchy scalp.

Natural cleansers wash away dirt and oil while five natural conditioners, including wheat germ protein, silk amino acids, and sunflower seed oil, strengthen and moisturize your hair. Unlike abrasive, 'medicated' shampoos, Melaleuca Original Shampoo® is gentle. It calms the scalp and softens the hair—without a burning sensation or strong odors—and is gentle enough for everyday use with all hair types and **by all ages**.

Suggested Weekly Hair Care Regimen

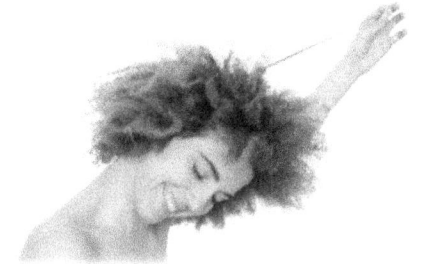

Pick a particular day of the week to shampoo and condition your hair. Let this be your regular day that you give attention to your hair. Use a natural organic shampoo (**without sodium laurel sulfate**); thoroughly wet hair while gently massaging your scalp by rotating it with the palm of your hand.

Shampoo your hair with emphasis on cleaning your scalp. DO NOT scratch your scalp—this will aggravate your problem; squeeze the shampoo throughout your hair strands and rinse hair thoroughly, moving your hair to expose your scalp and rinse very thoroughly making sure to rinse ALL the shampoo residue off your scalp.

Many times when the hair and scalp is not rinsed thoroughly, the residue from the shampoo and conditioner settles on to the scalp and can irritate an already sensitive scalp.

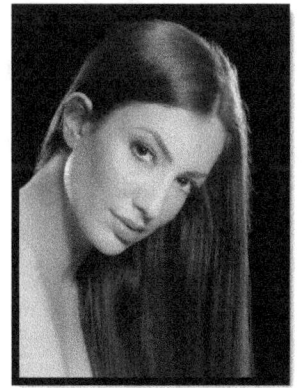

Add 5 – 10 drops of *Tea Tree Oil* to your conditioner and let the Tea Tree conditioner sit on your hair for about 10 -20 minutes. Rinse thoroughly and allow your hair to air-dry if possible, eliminating heat, which tends to dry your scalp. (Your hair may smell a little medicinal; it's okay though because it's only temporary—adding fragrance oil may irritate your scalp, so it's not suggested to use it).

Jojoba oil is excellent to drop onto your scalp to add moisture and luster to your hair.

Style your hair as usual but without any tension, pulling or stress on it.

Make sure to have a good attitude about this new process and think good thoughts. Believe it or not, your thoughts create *things* and a positive outlook can have a favorable affect.

PART 4

Natural Dandruff Treatments

Recipes, Herbs, and Other

Concoctions

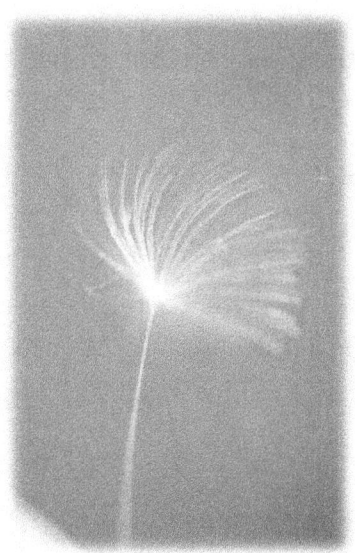

Natural Dandruff Treatments – Recipes, Herbs, and Other Concoctions

Because dandruff is a chronic condition the cause of which is still not completely established or agreed upon, the range of possible solutions that are claimed to work to treat the condition are almost endless.

Everyone who has ever suffered from dandruff (and remembers that one of the biggest anti-dandruff shampoo manufacturers, Procter & Gamble suggest that there are more dandruff sufferers than people who is completely dandruff free) has their own pet solution to the problem.

There are literally hundreds of these proposed solutions published all over the internet, some of which are likely to be far more effective than others. However, because each and every individual sufferer is different, it is not possible to suggest which of the treatments you are going to read about are likely to be most effective in any individual case.

Nevertheless, there are some of these treatments which are recommended on a wide variety of different sites, some of which are sites that have a good degree of authority (recognized medical sites, commonly used reference sites like about.com and eHow.com).

Consequently, these suggestions have been listed first, primarily because the fact that they appear on many different sites indicates that they work for many different people, whereas some of the other proposed solutions might be effective for far less people.

*The following remedy combinations can be prepared and poured into a spray bottle and sprayed directly onto the scalp.

Beetroot Juice

Juice one small 'beetroot' and add 1 tbsp. of vinegar

Mix vinegar and beetroot juice together before massaging it into the scalp, leaving in for 10 to 15 minutes and then rinsing the mixture out. Alternatively, a combination of juicing fresh ginger and beetroot juice can also be extremely effective; both of these roots – beetroot and ginger, have powerful antifungal qualities that can attack the yeast on your scalp which can lead to dandruff and this combination is effective in controlling dandruff.

Vinegar

Ever since man first discovered vinegar, it has been widely and commonly used for a great range of different medicinal purposes. It is extremely effective for dealing with dandruff, because it is rich in potassium and enzymes which will help to prevent an itchy scalp and dandruff.

There are many different ways you can use vinegar, as there are many different types of vinegar that you can use.

The first, most simple and basic way of using vinegar is to add just enough vinegar to cover the bottom of a bowl of warm water and gently rub the solution into your scalp(can also add solution to a spray bottle and spray onto your scalp) before retiring to bed for the night. Wrap your head in a towel to ensure that the solution does not evaporate or soak away into your pillow so that you can leave the solution on your head overnight (wear a plastic cap wrapped in a towel).

Do this every night for a couple of weeks, and you should start to notice a significant improvement in your dandruff situation.

Another suggestion is mixing four tablespoons of white vinegar together with two tablespoons of lemon juice. Gently massage the mixture into your scalp with your fingertips, once again trying to avoid contact between your fingernails and your scalp. Try to use a gentle circular rubbing motion, because this stimulates the blood flow to your scalp which also helps to minimize the likelihood of dandruff developing.

Leave the solution on for 30 minutes to one hour before washing it out with a gentle shampoo.

Incidentally, while you have probably tried medicated, anti-dandruff shampoos and you might even use them on a regular basis despite the possibility of adverse side-effects, you should try to **avoid combining** any of the natural remedies as suggested with a medicated shampoo for several reasons:

- **Firstly**, if you combine one of the natural solutions from above with medicated shampoo, and you see a significant improvement in your dandruff problem, it will be hard to isolate whether it is the natural solution or the medicated shampoo that has made the difference.

- **Secondly**, I haven't found any extensive research done into the possible reactions between medicated shampoos and the natural substances highlighted in this section. While this may not appear likely it should be a major concern, you have to remember that a substance like vinegar is extremely acidic, and therefore the possibility of some kind of chemical reaction between the chemicals in medicated shampoo and a vinegar-based solution cannot be completely eliminated.

Apple Cider Vinegar (ACV)

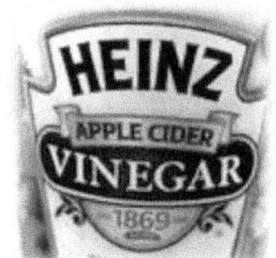

Apple cider vinegar is one particular variety of vinegar that has long been known to have significant health benefits, particularly in the realm of skin complaints.

This is because it is believed to stimulate blood circulation in the small capillaries just under the skin, plus it also has the ability to combat bacteria, viruses and the yeast that we have already established as one of the primary causes of dandruff (Malassezia). Furthermore, apple cider vinegar is rich in the alpha-hydroxyl acids that are known to help break down fatty, oily deposits on the skin, thereby reducing the amount of sebum on which the yeast that causes dandruff feeds.

As a topical treatment for dandruff, you can use apple cider vinegar diluted or undiluted.

- **Diluted:** add one-part vinegar to three parts warm water before gently massaging the solution into your scalp with exactly the same gentle circular rubbing motion as highlighted previously.
Leave the solution on your head for half to one hour before washing out with a gentle shampoo such as baby shampoo.

*Alternatively, for more severe cases of dandruff, you can use apple cider vinegar in the same way in its **undiluted** form.*

- Another method of using apple cider vinegar is to simply mix it with warm water as suggested a moment ago, spraying it onto your scalp with a spray bottle and gently massaging it in, taking care to avoid getting the solution in your eyes or ears. Once again, leave the solution on your head for an hour or so before gently washing it out.

Oatmeal

*Not recommended for those with kinky curly or loc'd hair

Another home-made dandruff treatment formulation that includes apple cider vinegar which you can easily create at home is as follows:

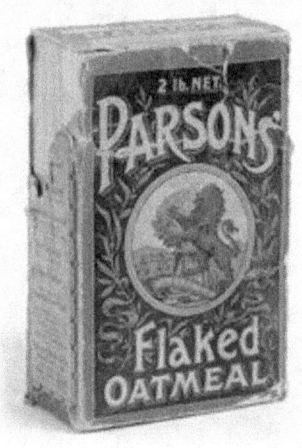

- Mix together one tablespoon of apple cider vinegar, two tablespoons of cornmeal or oatmeal and half a cup of grape seed oil. Mix oil together until you have a thick, coagulated paste and then apply the mixture to your scalp by gently massaging it in. Leave the mixture on your head for around one hour before rinsing out thoroughly and shampooing with a gentle, non-medicated shampoo such a as baby shampoo.

In this mixture, the apple cider vinegar does as it does in most cases, which is to balance the pH of your scalp, which is important, because in most dandruff sufferers, their scalp pH balance is skewed. On the other hand, the grape seed oil nourishes and soothes your skin, while the meal exfoliates the dead skin flakes.

As you can see, apple cider vinegar can be used in a wide variety of ways, with another option being nothing more complex than adding a few drops of vinegar to the final rinse you give your hair after washing it. As an alternative, add a few drops of lime or lemon juice to the final rinse, because once again, the acid nature of the fruit juice will destroy a significant percentage of the yeast on your scalp.

Tea Tree Oil

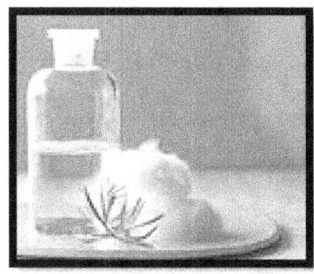 As suggested previously, although recent research has indicated that tea tree oil taken from the Melaleuca Alternifolia tree has potent antifungal and antibacterial qualities, this is a fact that the native peoples of Australia have known for many hundreds of years.

Although for many people tea tree oil shampoo is effective, it can be even more so if the oil is applied directly to the scalp, particularly if your dandruff is of the more serious or severe variety.

You can apply the oil several times a week by gently massaging it into your scalp and then leaving it on your hair for 30 minutes to one hour if at all possible.

Alternatively, buy the mildest non-medicated shampoo you can find (for example, baby shampoo), and mix the tea tree oil into the shampoo, using around 10 drops of oil for every eight fluid ounces of shampoo in the bottle.

Use this natural anti-dandruff shampoo in the same way that you would use ordinary shampoo, and you should see your dandruff problem reducing fairly rapidly.

Because of its antifungal qualities, tea tree oil is highly effective for minimizing the amount of yeast on your scalp, which in turn will do a great deal to minimize your dandruff as well.

Aloe Vera

Aloe Vera is another natural substance that has potent antifungal qualities, so applying the substance in gel form to your scalp is another

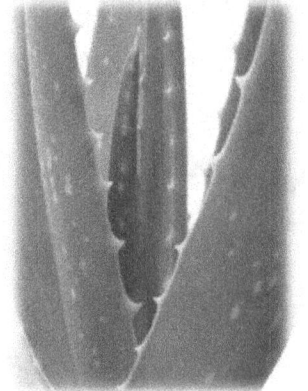 good way of reducing the amount of yeast on your scalp.

Another effective treatment is to buy Aloe Vera juice which you can drink to supplement your normal diet and rub it on your scalp. The juice contains many of the vitamins that you need in order to combat dandruff effectively, including vitamins A, B1, B6, B12 and vitamin E as well as folic acid.

Aloe Vera juice also contains 12 natural substances that have been shown to inhibit inflammatory conditions, and it helps to produce healthy skin as it provides a rich supply of collagen and elastin which repair and regenerate healthy skin.

In short, by drinking Aloe Vera juice as well as applying it topically to your scalp, you are fighting against your dandruff condition both internally and topically, which if nothing else should double your chances of successfully defeating your dandruff problem.

Olive Oil

Olive oil has been used for many centuries to combat a wide range of different medical conditions and it has long been recognized as an effective treatment for severe dandruff. Olive oil contains vitamin E and many other nutrients that are essential for healthy skin, so it is a solution that is worth trying.

Many sources suggest that olive oil becomes even more effective if it is mixed together in equal quantities with almond oil before the mixture is gently massaged into the scalp with the fingertips with gentle circular motions. The mixture should be left on for five to ten minutes, although if it starts to become uncomfortable or feel like it is beginning to burn (which seems to happen for a very small percentage of people who try this particular solution), you should wash it out immediately.

Otherwise, although the mixture might feel a little clammy or perhaps too oily while you are applying it, you should try to avoid washing it out until the mixture has completely dried out.

Jojoba Oil and its Benefits

Most people easily associate jojoba or jojoba oil with cosmetics. They 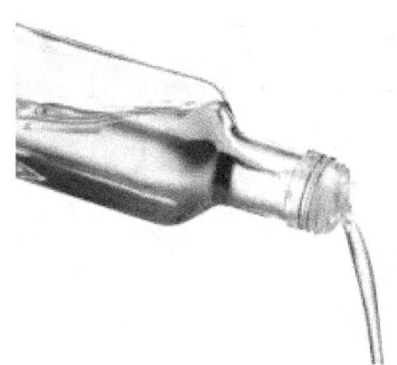 are used to seeing it in the products they use every day including moisturizers, shampoos and conditioners, even anti-aging and sun care products. But this hypoallergenic "oil" (actually a liquid wax) is also available in its simplest form, pure pressed jojoba oil, direct to consumers for their own personal use.

The amazing moisturizing properties of this unique seed oil have been known through the ages. Early Native Americans and the Indians who inhabited northwestern Mexico used the seeds and their oil for many applications. They found it useful in the making of a coffee-like beverage, medicines for cancer and kidney disorders, and chewing as a dietary supplement and an appetite suppressant when food was scarce; probably the most lasting use has been for treating skin and scalp issues.

First officially documented in 1822 by German botanist Johann Link and eventually renamed *Simmondsia chine sis* by Austrian botanist, Camillo Karl Schneider, in 1912, the unique properties of jojoba had been discovered by chemists in the 1930's. Traditionally, sperm whale oil had been the product of choice for use in cosmetics. But the 1971 U.S. ban on sperm whale oil import sent cosmetics manufacturers looking for a suitable replacement. Jojoba fit the bill.

Jojoba "oil" is different from other vegetable oils in that it is not actually triglyceride oil but a liquid wax. Its unique chemical makeup mimics the sebum naturally present on human skin. This is what makes it such a desirable product for the cosmetics we use every day.

According to the International Jojoba Export Council, jojoba is odorless, natural, non-greasy, and extremely stable. It doesn't break down when exposed to water or oxygen and, a natural carrier of Vitamin E and a natural antioxidant. It is an extremely efficient non-comedogenic moisture regulator, penetrating the skin to moisturize without blocking the pores.

A perennial woody shrub native to the semiarid Sonora Desert region of northwestern Mexico and the neighboring southwestern United States, jojoba grows in dense stands in the wild. It is presently also commercially cultivated in plantations all around the world in countries including Argentina, Australia, Chile, Egypt, Israel, Mexico, Peru, and the USA.

The seeds of the jojoba plant are crushed using various methods to extract the golden-yellow oil. It can be further processed with filtration to remove the color and odor. The forms most used by the cosmetics industry are "golden or refined (lite) jojoba, hydrogenated jojoba, jojoba esters, hydrolyzed jojoba, ethoxylated jojoba and other value added jojoba derivatives." (International Jojoba Export Council, www.ijec.net, *Manufacturing with Jojoba*)

Jojoba oil is readily available through many sources. While found in any number of commercial skin and hair care products, many suppliers provide various bottled quantities direct to the consumer at a reasonable price either through retail outlets or for purchase online.

The oil can be used topically, applied directly to the skin and scalp to remove makeup and product buildup, moisturize and soften rough, dry skin, even to relieve sunburn and condition and soothe skin during and after shaving. Added to other products like shampoos and liquid soaps, it aids in deep cleansing and conditioning. Mixing jojoba oil with your favorite essential oils makes for a relaxing, aromatic conditioning treatment for skin during massage.

A Few More Favorite Natural Dandruff Treatments - in brief

As suggested in the previous chapters, there are literally hundreds of different natural dandruff treatments that you will find detailed on a similarly large number of websites. The following list is intended to be a brief snapshot of many of these suggested methods that you might want to try also:

Apple tonic: Mix one tablespoon of apple juice/cider with three tablespoons of water and massage the mixture into your scalp three times a week.

Coconut oil and lemons: Massage warm pure coconut oil into your 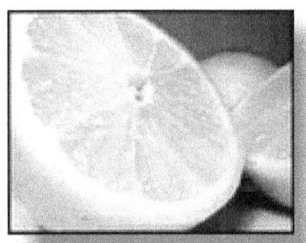 scalp and then rub in the juice of two lemons. Steam your hair by placing your head over a bowl of steaming hot water with the steam sealed in with a warm damp towel. After steaming for a few minutes, leave the mixture on your hair for a couple of hours before rinsing out, and repeat two or three times every week.

Thyme: Boil five heaped tablespoons of dried thyme in about a pint of water for a period of 10 to 15 minutes. After this, allow the infused liquid to cool before straining the thyme leaves out of the mixture and storing the resulting liquid in a jar. Keep in the fridge and massage the liquid into your scalp three or four times a week; rinse the solution out at least once a week.

Baking soda: It is now established that baking soda has powerful 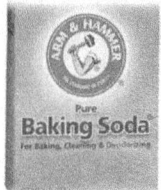 antifungal qualities, so making up a baking soda paste with warm water before applying it to your scalp should help to keep down the yeast which ultimately cause dandruff.

Winter melon or ash gourd: It is suggested on many Ayurveda medicine sites that grinding the seeds and skin of winter melon and then mixing them together with a little warm water before applying the mixture to the scalp can help to control dandruff. Once again, it appears that this mixture has powerful antifungal qualities so that it is effective for keeping yeast at bay. **(Not recommended for kinky curly or loc'd hair).**

Peanut oil and lemons: Mix the juice of half a lemon with eight teaspoons of peanut oil and rub the mixture into your hair. Leave the mixture on your scalp for 10 to 15 minutes before washing the solution away as normal.

Rosemary: Rosemary is the active ingredient in many commercial hair tonics and shampoo which rejuvenates the scalp and keeps the skin healthy. You may be able to buy rosemary oil in a health food shop, but if not, add eight tablespoons of dried rosemary to a pint of boiling water. Boil rosemary five minutes and then strain the used rosemary leaves. Apply the solution to your scalp and leave on your head for as long as possible. Rinse well.

Indian hemp: Indian hemp (also known as dogbane, wild cotton or Amy root) is a plant that can be found growing wild throughout North America that can be used to reduce dandruff. Simply crush the plant to extract the juice. Apply juice directly to the scalp. Leave in for an hour and then wash out of hair.

Scalp Scrub (gently): 2 TBS. Turbinado sugar, 5 -10 drops of tea tree oil, 2 TBS. Olive or Jojoba oil. Mix together and part hair, apply mixture sparingly and gently, massaging into scalp between parts in a circular manner all over head. Rinse well with lukewarm water, taking care to open hair and wash away residue completely. Allow hair to air dry and gently detangle hair with fingers.

Rosemary Hair Tonic Shampoo: 5 drops of rosemary essential oil, 5 drops of tea tree oil, 4 tsp. of non-fragranced shampoo. Mix well and shampoo hair as normal. Leave on hair about 5 minutes. Rinse well.

Essential Oil Skin Healing Recipe Blends

Note: following are a couple of *skin healing recipes* that you can try for skin problems. Mix carrier oils together with essential oils and massage into the skin--very soothing.

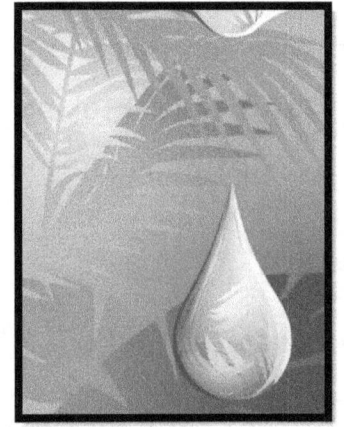

Eczema: 4 tsp. (carrier oil) - Olive, Jojoba or Almond oil; 4 drops of cedar wood essential oil, 4 drops of frankincense essential oil, 2 drops of lavender essential oil.

Ringworm: 4 drops of tea tree oil, 3 drops of sandalwood essential oil, 3 drops of lavender essential oil and 4 tsp. (carrier oil) - Olive, Jojoba or Almond oil.

Dermatitis: 4 tsp. (carrier oil) – Olive, Jojoba or Almond oil; 3 drops of palmarosa essential oil, 2 drops of roman chamomile essential oil.

Dermatitis: 4 tsp. (carrier oil) – Olive, Jojoba or Almond oil; 4 drops of lavender essential oil, 3 drops of tea tree oil, 3 drops of roman chamomile essential oil.

Psoriasis/Dermatitis/Eczema: 4 tsp. (carrier oil) – Olive, Jojoba or Almond oil; 3 drops of geranium essential oil, 3 drops of sandalwood essential oil, 4 drops of lavender essential oil.

Conclusion

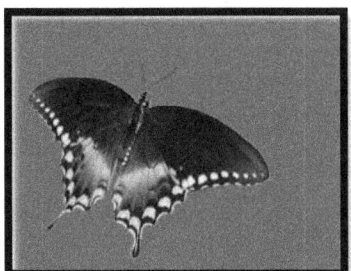

As you have no doubt gathered by now, there is no shortage of natural solutions for dandruff. *While none of these solutions can be presented as a complete cure*, many of the treatments that you have read in this book are extremely effective.

As with all medical conditions that require treatment, from the mildest to the most severe, there are natural solutions available for your dandruff problem that you should try *before* turning to chemical-based products.

While most of the chemical-based shampoos on the market have proved to be harmless for most users, there are a significant minority of people who suffer from dandruff for whom chemical-based shampoos are likely to make the problem worse rather than better. These are people who have particularly sensitive skin so the chemicals are more likely to aggravate their skin problems rather than help to clear them up.

However, even if you're not a person who suffers from overly sensitive skin, it still makes a great deal of sense to try natural solutions for your dandruff problem before turning to chemical-based shampoos, creams or potions, doesn't it? As suggested many times in this book, every individual dandruff sufferer is different so what works for one person will not necessarily work for another.

Nevertheless, there is no shortage of natural dandruff treatment choices available and I have attempted to highlight as many of the most effective natural dandruff treatments in this book as possible.

After reading this far, you should now have a far better understanding of what dandruff is, what causes it and how to treat it.

Consequently, you should, by now, consider lifestyle changes that can limit or minimize the outbreaks of dandruff that you will suffer subsequently before gaining knowledge about the information contained in this book.

As you have come to discover, dandruff is a problem that is fully controllable and curable (in many cases). I hope you appreciate by now, it is **NOT** necessary to live with the annoyance of dandruff without doing something about it…naturally.

To combat dandruff is not that difficult or complex, and armed with the knowledge that you now have, there is no reason to tolerate your dandruff for one moment longer.

Glossary of Terms

Hair=Hair is quite simply defined as a form of protein called Keratin

Sebum=an oily secretion of the sebaceous glands

Malassezia=Malassezia is a lipophilic fungal genus, members of which are part of the normal human scalp flora. M. restricta and M. globosa feed on lipids secreted from the hair follicles. The partially digested lipids that linger on the skin cause the familiar irritation of the scalp that leads to dandruff.

Scalp flora=The skin flora is composed of a large number of microorganisms which are found between the hair follicles and the sweat pores that cover the surface of the skin

Melaleuca Alternifolia=Tea tree oil can kill bacteria and fungi. It comes from the evergreen leaves of the Australian Melaleuca Alternifolia tree

Gamma Linolenic Acid=Gamma linolenic acid is a fatty substance found in various plant seed oils such as borage oil and evening primrose oil. People use it as medicine.
 Gamma linolenic acid (GLA) is used for conditions that affect the skin including systemic sclerosis, psoriasis, and eczema

Isoflavones=Isoflavones are polyphenolic compounds that are capable of exerting estrogen-like effects

Melatonin=a hormone secreted by the pineal gland that inhibits melanin formation and is thought to be concerned with regulating the reproductive cycle

Pineal gland=a pea-sized conical mass of tissue behind the third ventricle of the brain, secreting a hormone like substance in some mammals

Olfactory receptors=expressed in the cell membranes of olfactory receptor neurons are responsible for the detection of odor molecules.

Encephalin=either of two compounds that occur naturally in the brain. They are peptides related to the endorphins, with similar physiological effects

Potassium=the chemical element of atomic number 19, a soft silvery-white reactive metal of the alkali metal group; Potassium is a mineral that, among other things, helps your muscles contract, helps regulate fluids and mineral balance in and out of body cells and helps maintain normal blood pressure by blunting the effect of sodium

Enzymes=a substance produced by a living organism that acts as a catalyst to bring about a specific biochemical reaction; enzymes mostly assist in the metabolic reactions of cells such as respiration, digestion and photosynthesis

Alpha hydroxyl acid=an organic acid containing a hydroxyl group bonded to the carbon atom adjacent to the carboxylic acid group. A number of such compounds are used in skin-care preparations for their exfoliating properties

Collagen=the main structural protein found in animal connective tissue, yielding gelatin when boiled

Elastin=an elastic, fibrous glycoprotein found in connective tissue

Sodium Laureth/Lauryl Sulfate= is an anionic detergent; is an inexpensive and very effective foaming agent. ...Sodium lauryl sulfate is a surfactant, detergent, and emulsifier used in thousands of cosmetic products, as well as in industrial cleaners. It is present in nearly all shampoos, scalp treatments, hair color and bleaching agents, toothpastes, body washes and cleansers, make-up foundations, liquid hand soaps, laundry detergents, and bath oils/bath salts. Although SLS originates from coconuts, the chemical is anything but natural. The real problem with SLES/SLS is that the manufacturing process (ethoxylation) results in SLES/SLS being contaminated with 1, 4 dioxane, a carcinogenic by-product.

Sodium Chloride=Sodium chloride—also known as salt

Cetyl Alcohol=a waxy alcohol occurring in feces and esterified in spermaceti and wool wax. It is used in cosmetics and as an emulsifier

Hydrochloric Acid=is a clear, colorless, highly pungent solution of hydrogen chloride (HCl) in water. It is a highly corrosive, strong mineral acid with many industrial uses. Hydrochloric acid is found naturally in gastric acid

Butylated Hydroxytoluene=a synthetic antioxidant used to preserve fats and oils in foods, medicinal drugs, and cosmetics

Propylene Glycol=a liquid alcohol that is used as a solvent, in antifreeze, and in the food, plastics, and perfume industries

Beautiful Hair Products

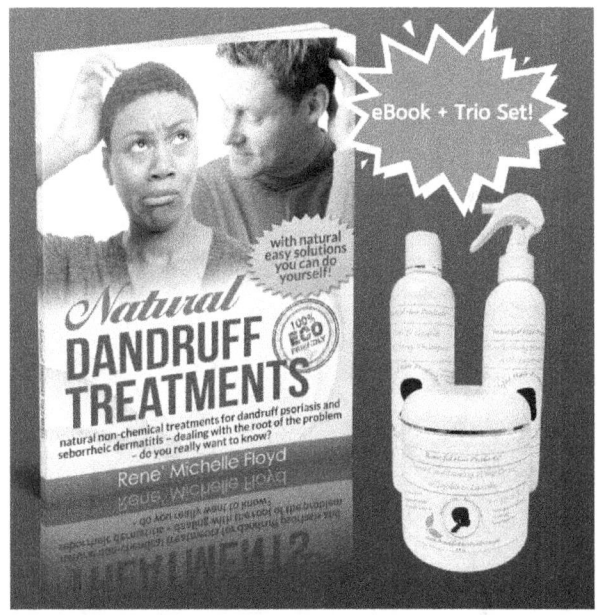

- Beautiful Hair Super Conditioning Whip Crème w/Jojoba Oil & Lanolin—8 oz. jar
- Moisturizing Hair Spray—8 oz.
- Pure & Gentle Clarifying Shampoo—8 oz.
- Natural Dandruff Treatments book—100+ pages!

MORE PRODUCTS TO COME!!

**For more information on how to treat dandruff naturally and how to purchase *Natural Green Products* contact René Michelle Floyd directly at: (951) 567-6259 or directly via email: Rene@BeautifulHairProducts.com

We are very social so let's stay connected

BHP Store: http://www.BeautifulHairProducts.com

- **Tweet Us**: http://www.Twitter.com/BHPhair

- **Facebook us**:
  https://www.facebook.com/BeautifulHairProducts/

- **Instagram:**
  http://www.Instagram.com/BeautifulHairProducts

- **Watch Us**: http://youtube.com/ReneMFloyd

- **Link to Us**: http://LinkedIn.com/in/ReneMichelleFloyd

~RESOURCES~

*All links to the *Resources* are in the back of this book*

Book: Body Ecology Diet by Donna Gates

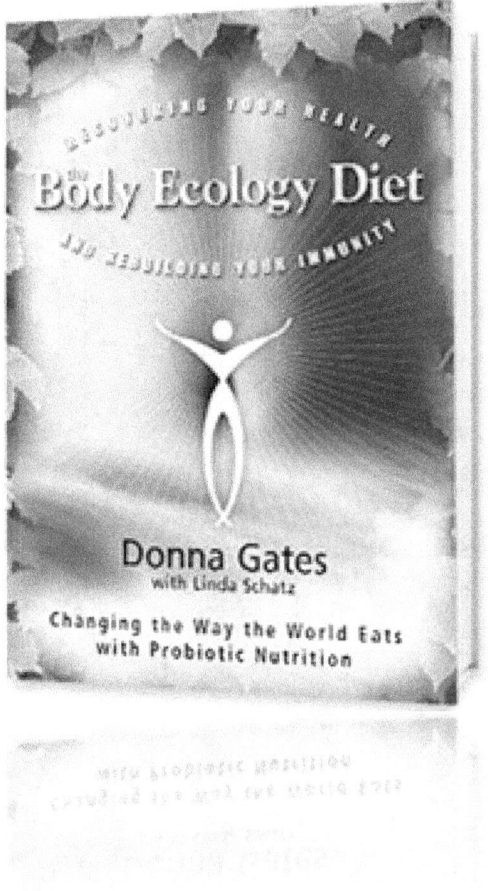

The Body Ecology Diet website has a wealth of information. You will find a host of information on Enema's and vitamin and mineral supplementation. Check out their website. I encourage you to purchase the book and take advantage of their selection of Super foods and Educational materials. A great place to shop for everything you need to get you on the road to health and healing.

A Book about Curing Psoriasis

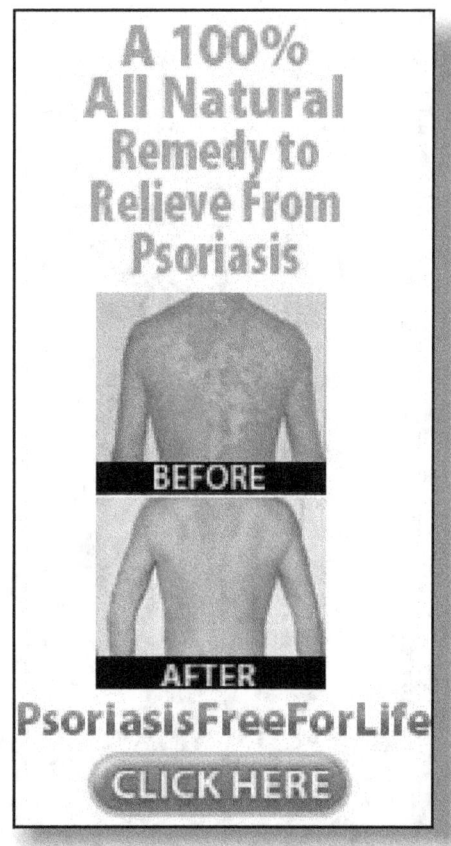

Psoriasis Free for Life by Katie Wilson, an Alternative Medical Practitioner and Researcher, has helped so many people I just had to share the website with you. Check the website out and read the testimonies of those who've been helped; not only do you get the Psoriasis Free for Life secrets, but you get seven (7) more books as a bonus and she offers a 60 day guarantee or your money back. You have nothing to lose. Go see what it can possibly do for you.

One of a Kind Vegetarian Cookbook

AND

The Divine Weight Loss Formula

By Barbara L. Ray

Two books in one!

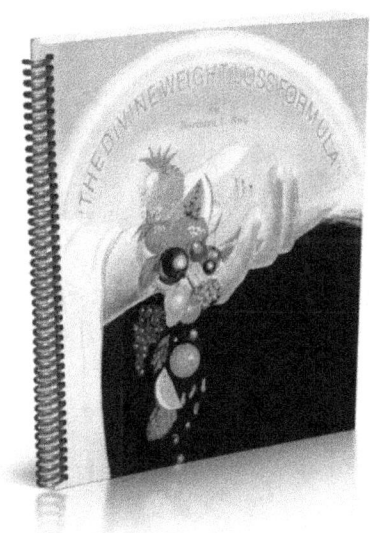

One of A Kind Vegetarian Cookbook AND The Divine Weight Loss Formula by Barbara L. Ray (Health Consultant and Vegan) is a combined edition! Two books in one! Filled with delicious vegetarian recipes and fresh juice recipes that is simple and easy to make. A great book for those desiring to transition into a more healthy way of cooking...you will find a food plan and menu included...of course, a healthy head of hair is directly linked to the diet you eat and the liquid you drink...very informative and simple. OKVC and TDWLF book is *a must!*

Please Leave Your Review on Amazon.com

Thank you so much for choosing my book to read. I hope this book met your expectations. If NDT was helpful to you, can you do me a favor? **Please** leave your review for this book on my author page at Amazon.com.

My author page is: http://www.amazon.com/Rene-Michelle-Floyd/e/B006EU0K4Q

Simply visit my author page, click on the title of the book you're leaving a review for and scroll halfway down the page to where it says '**write a customer review**', click and type in your review.

Your review is greatly appreciated. It helps the work get discovered by many others who are looking for answers just like you.

Please tell your friends and family about this book. Your promotion is needed and I thank you in advance for your kindness.

RESOURCES LINKS

Beautiful Hair Products

Beautiful Hair Products are made from natural and organic ingredients which include: fresh handmade to order- conditioner and moisturizing hair spray- free of harmful chemicals that strip and damage the hair. *Especially delicious for natural hair, Dreadlocks, Sisterlocks(tm), Braids, Twists, and Brotherlocks–you name it!*

http://BeautifulHairProducts.com

Vegetarian and Weight Loss Cookbook

One of A Kind Vegetarian Cookbook AND The Divine Weight Loss Formula by Barbara L. Ray (Health Consultant and Vegan) is a combined edition! Two books in one! Filled with delicious vegetarian recipes and fresh juice recipes that is simple and easy to make. A great book for those desiring to transition into a healthier way of cooking.

http://amzn.to/2x4Z1r8

Vitamin and Mineral Supplements

Balanced mineral supplements that deliver detox benefits, increase immune system, increase metabolism and improve heart health.

https://bodyecology.com/355-18.html

Bowel and Enema Health

Cleansing nutritional supplements to nourish and heal your inner ecosystem with alkalizing ingredients to rebuild the health of your intestines for weight control and body detoxification.

https://bodyecology.com/355-17.html

Psoriasis Free for Life by Katie Wilson

The root cause of psoriasis is NOT a skin disease. It's an immune system disease. And when you learn how to help boost your immunity and control outbreaks, you'll not only be symptom free but psoriasis free as well!

http://femineen.psoriasis.hop.clickbank.net

[Video] Natural Dandruff Treatments book and the benefits of Tea Tree Oil and Natural Shampoo for dandruff and other scalp issues

http://www.youtube.com/watch?v=xHaloMd8mIM&feature=youtu.be

Learning Yoga

Through the practice of Yoga, you can develop internal defenses to protect the mind and body. The benefits are numerous and a daily practice will help you enjoy many of them.

Deep Breathing

'Breath is life.' So the saying goes, and author Dennis Lewis expands the listener's awareness of the powerful health benefits of full breath. Breathing has not only a physical dimension, but also a metaphysical and spiritual one. Just as there is a personal aspect to breath, there is a communal one, as we all share the same oxygen with everyone who has ever lived.

Jeanne Rose

Jeanne Rose is the founder of New Age Creations, the first body-care company in the United States to use aromatherapy (since 1967). She is the Director of the Institute of Aromatic Studies, principal tutor of both the Herbal Studies Course and the Aromatherapy Studies Course - Practitioner by home-study. She brings 40 years of experience and personal research in her practice of Aromatherapy.

http://www.jeannerose.net/

The Health Risks & Benefits of the Oleander Plant

Known in ancient texts as "the desert rose," historical references show that 15th century B.C. Mesopotamians trusted in the healing benefits of oleander extracts. From a remedy for hangovers to an herb studied for cancer, the Babylonians, Romans, Arabs and ancient Greeks alike used this herbal extract for a variety of health concerns.

http://www.globalhealingcenter.com/natural-health/oleander/

15 Big Benefits of Water by Jennifer Goldstein

I came across this wonder article about the benefits of water in regards to the health of your hair. Whether you want shinier hair, younger skin, a healthier body (or all three!), pure, clear water is the world's best beauty elixir.

http://www.health.com/health/gallery/0,,20396298,00.html

Let's Go Amazon.com Shopping!!

*All the following links will take you directly to the pages where you will find the **exact** recommended products found in this book. I am an affiliate of these products. If you purchase a product, I will get a *small* commission for referring these wonderful products to you. Any little bit helps. Thank you in advance for your support * Peace *

Jojoba Oil

- Pure uncut cold pressed jojoba oil
- Keep the skin moist and wrinkle free.
- Imparts relief to dehydrated and ultra-sensitive skin.
- It reduces skin inflammation and helps in curing several skin disorders such as eczema and psoriasis.

http://amzn.to/2xi0pG5

Tea Tree Oil (Melaleuca Alternifolia)

Tea Tree Oil has been a part of Australia's Aboriginal culture for thousands of years based on its powerful cleansing properties. Today, it is commonly used in a number of cosmetic and beauty applications. NOW® Tea Tree Oil is 100% pure, steam-distilled from the leaves of Melaleuca Alternifolia, and mixes well with many other essential oils.

http://amzn.to/2yazGZo

Black Currant Oil

- Each soft gel contains almost double the GLA content of evening primrose oil
- Black currant oil is derived from the ribesnigrum plant better known as black currant
- It regulates the menstrual cycle and premenstrual syndrome in women

http://amzn.to/2xNMY1O

Evening (Super) Primrose Oil

NOW® Super Primrose Oil is a high potency Evening Primrose (EPO) supplement containing naturally occurring Gamma Linoleic Acid (GLA). GLA is a fatty acid that is important for healthy inflammatory and immune response. Evening Primrose Oil may be used to provide nutritional support for mild discomfort associated with PMS. Evening Primrose Oil also helps maintain healthy skin and circulatory function.* NOW® Super Primrose is hexane free

http://amzn.to/2yap3pA

Apple Cider Vinegar

Certified Bragg Organic Raw Apple Cider Vinegar is unfiltered, unheated and unpasteurized. Aged in wood, this Apple Cider Vinegar is a wholesome way to add a delicious flavor to most foods, salads, veggies and even popcorn

http://amzn.to/2xhtWPX

Shea Moisture Baby Shampoo

Soothing Aloe Vera skin-softening Argan oil and healing chamomile, frankincense & myrrh extracts cleanse and nourish baby's delicate hair and body. Shea Butter: Deeply moisturizes and heals dry skin with its high content of fatty acids and vitamins Argan oil: High in vitamin E, this rare oil softens and renews the skin With frankincense & myrrh: Given as a gift of beauty throughout history, these precious extracts repair and rejuvenate skin Suitable for all ages No parabens, phthalates, paraffin, gluten, propylene glycol, mineral oil, synthetic fragrance, PABA, synthetic color, DEA, or sulfates Cruelty free, no animal testing Made in USA

http://amzn.to/2ffKAJO

Aloe Vera Gel

Aloe Vera Juice Organic Whole Leaf No Preservatives by Lily Of The Desert 32 oz. Liquid Aloe Vera Juice Organic Whole Leaf No Preservatives 32 oz. Liquid Product Enjoy all the 200 biologically active components of our Regular Aloe Vera Juices minus the preservatives. Our Preservative Free Aloe Vera Juice delivers essential amino acids vitamins minerals and enzymes

http://amzn.to/2wrkXNA

Essential Oils

Blends Include- Calming (Lemongrass, Sweet Orange & Ylang Ylang), Four Thieves (Cinnamon, Clove, Eucalyptus, Lemon & Rosemary), Hope (Cassia, Lemongrass, Rosemary, Sweet Orange & Tangerine), Meditation (Clary Sage, Frankincense, Patchouli, Sweet Orange, Thyme & Ylang Ylang), Purification (Eucalyptus, Grapefruit, Lemon, Lemongrass & Lime), Stay Alert (Eucalyptus, Lavender, Peppermint & Pine) and Stress Relief (Bergamot, Blood Orange, Grapefruit, Patchouli & Ylang Ylang)

http://amzn.to/2yafoQ0

Coconut Oil

This organic, unrefined Coconut Oil is ideal for hair and body care. It provides a protective layer to combat the damaging effects of sun, wind and cold weather. Use it to restore soft, smooth skin and hair. So pure, you can eat it. Enjoy its rich, natural tropical scent!

http://amzn.to/2yaEBtA

Olive Oil

First cold-pressed extra virgin oil Manufactured in Italy Makes for an ideal gift Partanna Extra Virgin Olive Oil has a fruity taste. It gives you a peppery flavor and the true essence of Italy in each pack. This herbaceous is canned to lock the flavor. Just open the tin and use it as you like.

http://amzn.to/2xM3ZcL

Nit Comb (for picking out Lice & their eggs)

Nit Free TERMINATOR Comb is the ultimate Tool to fight Head Lice and their eggs (nits). ANTI-SLIP BANDS allow for better gripping and control. ADVANCED LASER TECHNOLOGY welding makes the comb sturdy and long-lasting. MICROGROOVED TEETH consist of micro spirals around the teeth that allow the teeth to grip the eggs and lice pulling them freely from the hair. The Nit Free Terminator comb is the leading comb on the market backed by university case studies. The #1 comb used by professional nit pickers.

http://amzn.to/2ffb9i2